HEALTH
PROFESSIONALS
STYLEBOOK

HEALTH PROFESSIONALS STYLEBOOK

PUTTING YOUR LANGUAGE TO WORK

Shirley H. Fondiller, EdD, RN

Barbara J. Nerone, APR

National League for Nursing Press • New York
Pub. No. 14-2551

Copyright © 1993
National League for Nursing Press
350 Hudson Street, New York, NY 10014

ISBN 0-88737-603-7

The views expressed in this publication represent the views of the authors and do not necessarily reflect the official views of the National League for Nursing.

This book was set in Palatino by Publications Development Company of Texas.

The editor and designer was Maryan Malone.

Automated Graphic Systems was the printer and binder.

Cover design by Lauren Stevens.

Printed in the United States of America.

". . . the most thorough knowledge of human nature, the happiest delineation of its varieties, the liveliest effusions of wit and humour are conveyed to the world in the best chosen English."

Jane Austen
Northanger Abbey

About the Authors

Shirley H. Fondiller, EdD, RN, an internationally known journalist, educator, and historian, is cofounder and principal of Publishing for Health Dimensions (*phd*), an editorial service for nurses and health professionals. She is an adjunct associate professor at Teachers College, Columbia University. Her most recent work is *The Writer's Workbook* (1992), a hands-on resource for beginning authors in the health field. She also has written monographs for leading private foundations, historiographies of influential national organizations, and scripts for the broadcast media.

Barbara J. Nerone, APR, has a broad background in the communications field. She has written and edited articles for nursing journals as well as publications of national associations and service agencies. Elected to the Counselors' Academy of the Public Relations Society of America, she is cofounder and principal of Publishing for Health Dimensions (*phd*).

Preface

You have been learning how to write since you began going to school, or perhaps before. Along the way, you probably studied many composition primers to enhance your communication skills in both the spoken and written word. If you were lucky, one of your early treasures was the classic Warriner grammar, whose basics on English composition apply more than ever. Go back and read it from cover to cover, whether for the first time or the fifth—but never the last.

Writing is a craft that must be cultivated. When your writing is clear and purposeful, your audience will want more and will read on. To captivate that reader from the outset will depend not only on your topic but on how well you can express yourself.

Nurses and other health professionals are fortunate in having limitless opportunities for sharing their experiences. Flourishing journal and book markets are craving more and better works about clinical practice, education, management, health policy, research, and so on. You will want to join other successful writers in your profession. And why not? You have lots of ideas just waiting to be put into print. But there's the rub. Jotting down those ideas and organizing them in a literate and interesting fashion are not always easy.

Your concern about the process is indeed justified. As an indication of publishers' efforts to help stylebooks have appeared increasingly in recent years. Many of these books are excellent guides, particularly for general principles. Yet, there are obvious gaps in the specific information you need for communicating in your area. Face it: Health professionals have a language all their own!

This *Stylebook* is based to a large extent on our direct contact with faculty, students, clinicians, administrators, and others eager to perfect their prose. From their writings, we have culled the more serious and recurring problems.

Bear in mind that this manual will not write an essay or paper for you, but it will provide valuable suggestions on proper usage and style. In this way, it will help you to be your own editor and to cut down on excessive rewrite. Although not a text on the writing process or on tips for approaching an editor successfully, it can act as a catalyst propelling you into the publishing arena. If you are a student, the *Stylebook* will greatly benefit your writing of term papers, theses, and dissertations. Practitioners in the work environment will learn how to refine their writing skills to generate succinct and solid documentation.

The art of speaking and writing well should be the aim of all health professionals. By perfecting your use of language, you will be able to articulate your thoughts more clearly. Whether your job involves such tasks as writing reports and memorandums, preparing papers and published works, or presenting scholarly addresses or informal talks, this *Stylebook* will be an indispensable resource.

Shirley H. Fondiller, EdD, RN
Barbara J. Nerone, APR

Acknowledgments

We extend our appreciation to the many colleagues, clients, and students whose persistent pleas for a book of this nature stimulated our call to action. Once into the effort, numerous consultants helped in moving the book along.

In particular, we wish to acknowledge Keith Bradkowski, clinical nursing director of surgery at Cedars-Sinai Medical Center in Los Angeles, for keeping us au courant with the abbreviations and acronyms in the practice area. For her editorial expertise, we are grateful to Dorothy Nayer, a seasoned adviser to health professionals.

Another person deserving recognition is Donna Reid, copy chief at the *American Journal of Nursing*. A special word of gratitude goes to Fred Pattison, director of the Sophia Palmer Library of the American Journal of Nursing Company, who graciously made available some excellent resources. In addition, we appreciate the assistance of Mary Anne Rizzolo, director of videodisc development, AJN Company, for her timely information on computer programming.

Finally, we would like to thank Allan Graubard, editorial director of the National League for Nursing, for his wise counsel and infinite patience throughout the course of the project.

S.H.F.
B.J.N.

Foreword

Learn to write well, or not to write at all.

JOHN DRYDEN

Today, perhaps more than ever, health professionals must be concerned with communication. Being able to communicate clearly and effectively—especially through writing—can make the difference in getting your ideas across and having an impact. Clear and effective communication has become increasingly important, whether in the context of clinical practice, scholarship that attempts to communicate new ideas or report research findings to colleagues, or articulating policy to the broader public. Writing that has clarity of purpose and is well-organized and compelling will not only be read but will speak with authority.

There is an old adage that writing tends to beget more writing, and more writing begets better writing. My experience tells me that this is true. But good writing is not easy to achieve. It demands much more than simply rewriting. Good writing—the best writing—requires of the writer not only a thorough command of his or her subject or an idea that is worth communicating to others, but also skills that can be learned and mastered. Above all, good writing requires a working knowledge of the fundamental mechanics of language, complexities of syntax, elements of style, and principles of proper usage.

To this end, the *Health Professionals Stylebook—Putting Your Language to Work* is a remarkably useful book. It provides a complete guide to writing and offers precisely the kind of guidance on style and usage that health professionals—whether inexperienced writers or seasoned authors—will appreciate.

What makes this stylebook unique?

First, it has been written with the special needs of health professionals in mind. Second, it is designed to be used in conjunction with generic style manuals and other writing guides. Third, Shirley H. Fondiller and Barbara J. Nerone are recognized experts in the field of professional communication. In concept and attention to detail, the *Stylebook* reflects the combined insight of their many years of experience as leading authors, editors, and journalists.

Whether you are a student, clinician, administrator, or scientist in any of the health professions, the *Stylebook* should be an invaluable resource in helping you to improve your writing. And whether you write with pen or at the keyboard, this promises to be an essential little book, one that should never be too far from your desk.

John P. Allegrante, PhD
Professor of Health Education
and Director
Division of Health Services, Sciences,
and Education
Teachers College
Columbia University
New York, New York

Introduction:
About the *Stylebook*

Many people have difficulty expressing themselves, largely because of inadequate or faulty preparation in composition in their early years. Unless they are prolific readers, they need to acquire some understanding of basic grammatical terms, constructions, and stylistic devices. By presenting some of the fundamental concepts on the use of language, this *Stylebook,* targeted to health professionals, aims to encourage them to write more effectively.

Whereas grammar describes the system of language, syntax is the way in which you put words together to form phrases, clauses, or sentences. When you study usage, your concern is with the appropriate form of expression. The guide consists of several sections that deal with the conventions of language and proper application. Through example, it will show you how to substitute the more acceptable forms of usage in place of the common, everyday words and phrases that undermine your writing. By practicing the proper techniques, you will learn to accentuate the substance and eliminate the "fluff."

As a motivator, the book will help you to develop your own style—an elusive quality to describe, but one highly individualized because it reflects your personality and your *Weltanschauung.* No one said it better than E. B. White when he characterized style as the sound a writer's words make on paper. Strunk and White's (1979) diminutive manual has more wisdom than many of the more expansive texts now available. Always keep it within reach!

In planning for the present guide, our approach was to examine existing stylebooks for their relevance, cull or modify what was particularly useful, and add information for health professionals not found elsewhere. We knew that some duplication would be inevitable but for emphasis only.

At the outset of our mission, we began a scrupulous search of contemporary style manuals of prominent news and news gathering organizations, professional associations, universities, and journal and book publishers. Our faithful companions throughout the investigative and writing phases included a host of general, medical, and nursing dictionaries as well as old and new texts on English composition and style.

One of the most difficult though challenging aspects of the effort was not merely selecting the entries, but determining the appropriate descriptions and examples. This was no easy task in light of the differing suggestions and contradictory views that appeared in many of the reference materials. In some instances, the differences seemed valid, indicating only a question of preference. The *Stylebook* has supported this flexibility.

Other situations occurred, however, in which we deliberately became arbitrary in determining usage. A case in point was the sequence of academic degrees and professional titles after a person's surname. We strongly concurred with the experts from the *New York Times* and Associated Press, who recommend that academic degrees *precede* the professional designation, as in: Belinda Farr, PhD, RN. We believe this represents the best or preferred form.

Dictionaries also proved to be invaluable resources. Writers need to familiarize themselves with the kinds of information contained in dictionaries—particularly the newer editions—and what each offers. In our search, we discovered that although dictionaries varied in the number of entries and methods of presenting information, many reported on the use of language.

Our dictionary of choice was *Webster's New World College Dictionary* (1989) because of its precision and clarity. The latest edition of *The American Heritage Dictionary of the English Language* (1992) was helpful because of its expanded description in the usage area. At the same time, we found ambiguity in some of the entries. Readers were left to ponder the preferred choice. The dictionary's panel of experts described words such as *prioritize* and *privatize* as corporate or bureaucratic jargon but did not suggest eliminating them as it had done in the previous editions.

The panel's recent advice was to use the words "with caution until they have passed the test of manifest utility and acceptance by reputable writers" (p. 959). Consistent with other sources, however, we were more firm in recommending that in professional writing, questionable words should be avoided until and if they become recognized as part of the language.

What You Can Expect

The first section, which discusses usage, offers an alphabetical listing of entries, frequently followed by examples applicable to nurses and other health professionals. We did not intend to define all words and phrases, but some definitions were necessary to convey the usage more clearly. The first draft of the manuscript included several words that were shifted later to other categories. In most situations, the names of individuals cited in the examples were meant to be fictitious. Throughout the section, the terms "professional writing" and "formal writing" have been used interchangeably, as have the verbs "capitalize" and "uppercase."

The book covers American usage only, as reflected in the descriptions and spellings of words and phrases. Other nations have their own writing style preferences. A common error occurs in this country when writers spell words like *acknowledgment* with an extra "e" (*acknowledgement*). The latter choice may be the correct form in Great Britain or Canada, but it should not appear in American writing. British spellings also differ in other ways, such as in converting words like *organization* into *organisation*. An awareness of language conventions adopted by other lands is not only illuminating but beneficial for communicators as our world becomes smaller.

The section on abbreviations and acronyms developed into an extremely complex undertaking. With the advent of new technology, procedures, and protocols in American health care, new terminology has evolved. In Part A of this section, we tried to capture most of these changes. In Part B, which included nursing and health-related organizations, it was not feasible to list all the groups in light of their extensive number. The entries selected should be helpful in identifying the abbreviations and acronyms of well-known groups in the field. Fortunately, other sources carry excellent directories, such as those published by the American Hospital Association and the *American Journal of Nursing*. The annual April issue of the *AJN* has a complete listing of the names and addresses of nursing organizations, as well as some abbreviations.

Subsequent sections of the *Stylebook* focus on wordage and its many facets. You may even be dazzled a little by the flagrant use of poor practices that deter rather than foster good writing. Undoubtedly, you will recognize many of the overworked and extra words, the interminable clichés, and the jargon of the trade. You may even be convinced to become more circumspect after studying this compendium of excessive wordiness.

In Section VIII, we urge you to observe carefully the list of correctly spelled words that have appeared frequently and repeatedly as misspellings in manuscripts, memorandums, reports, scholarly papers, and similar written material. If you want to earn "brownie points" with journal and book editors, employers, colleagues, and others who will read your work, watch out for careless spellings.

At the end of the manual is *your* reference guide, selected with care and studied diligently. The citations represent what we consider the best in the writing business. They will be particularly helpful in providing you with supplementary information to the *Health Professionals Stylebook*.

Summary

As the world of health care continues to expand, so will its language. Who ever heard of DRGs or case management a few decades ago? In the present work, we have tried to cite the most useful entries, hoping that there are no serious omissions. The selections as well as their interpretations have undergone rigorous review by knowledgeable health professionals and editorial experts.

In time, this book will undergo change. We invite you as representatives of the health care community and communicators in your respective fields to share with us your comments and suggestions for new areas of need. In the meantime, however, put *your* language to work!

Contents

I

Understand Usage—What It's All About

A

a, an.   Indefinite articles. Use a before words beginning with a consonant or consonant sound: *a nurse, a hospital, a procedure.* Use an before words beginning with a vowel sound: *an unknown origin, an inoperable tumor.* The use of a and an before abbreviations or numbers depends on the sound: *an NYU student, an IV, a two-step procedure, an eight-hour shift.*

Words beginning with h, when the initial h is not pronounced, are preceded by an.

Dr. Bond indicated that the therapy session would last an hour.

A word with an h firmly emphasized in the first syllable is preceded by a and not an.

Her paper focused on a history of postanesthesia recovery rooms.

Adjectives such as historic, historical, and habitual are generally preceded by an although they can be preceded by a.

Bette preferred a historical novel to an inflated autobiography.

<u>abbreviations, acronyms</u>.   (See also Section II.) An <u>abbreviation</u> is a shortened form of a word or phrase used chiefly in writing to represent the complete form.

RN	*registered nurse*
ANA	*American Nurses Association*
DRG	*Diagnostic Related Group*

Spell out a proper name or word the first time it is mentioned. Then use the abbreviation or acronym. In most cases, it is not necessary to insert the abbreviation in parenthesis following the proper name the first time it is written, unless the abbreviation might be misunderstood.

Elliot had suffered a myocardial infarction in 1990. He hoped that it would be his only MI.

The American Nurses Association supports . . . . ANA also works toward . . . .

Be careful when using the same abbreviation for two different titles. For example, AACN is the abbreviation for both the American Association of Critical Care Nurses <u>and</u> the American Association of Colleges of Nursing. In such <u>cases</u>, spell out the proper name to avoid possible misunderstanding.

An <u>acronym</u> is a word formed with the first letter or letters of each of a series of words, such as *W.H.O.* for *World Health Organization* and *radar* for *radio detecting and ranging*.

Do not use a period between the letters of the acronym or abbreviation, except when they spell a word that might be misunderstood or when the acronym or abbreviation has another meaning. Examples are:

W.H.O.	*World Health Organization*
N.O.W.	*National Organization for Women*
W.A.C.	*Women's Army Corps*
I.N.A.N.E.	*International Academy of Nursing Editors*

academic degrees.   Use abbreviations such as MS or DNSc only after a full name and never after a last name appearing alone. The trend is to omit periods in abbreviations of academic degrees. Be consistent if you wish to use them.

Academic degrees should precede professional titles. Some publications, however, reverse the order.

Eleanor Drake, PhD, RN (more acceptable form)

Eleanor Drake, RN, PhD

The MD (doctor of medicine) and PhD (doctor of philosophy) are academic degrees. When both are stated, the order is determined by the first earned degree.

Jeremy Welby, MD, PhD (if Dr. Welby earned his MD first)

An honorary doctorate is not an earned degree and therefore should not be listed as a credential after an individual's name. Also, do not refer to a person with an honorary degree as "Doctor," unless the individual already has an earned doctorate.

Although the BA, BS, and BSN are earned degrees, do not use them in a listing of credentials when followed by an advanced degree. The bachelor's degree is assumed.

Sara Scott, MA, RN

The above principle applies to the master's degree when a doctoral degree has been earned. Exceptions occur when degrees have been earned in different disciplines, such as when a PhD nurse also has an MBA.

Lucie Anderson, MBA, PhD, RN

Although it is common practice in nursing to use the BS and BSN along with the RN in bylines, as well as in references, such use rarely occurs in other disciplines. An English major or an engineer, for example, would <u>never</u> use:

Mark Cummings, BA, director of sales, Columbia Computer Corporation

For the correct attribution on a manuscript, check the format of the publication in which you wish to publish.

academic and other titles.
 a. *academic titles.* Capitalize when used before a person's name. Use lower case (and set off with commas) after a name. Capitalize a school or college name, when used alone or identified with a university, but lowercase academic departments or divisions.

> *Dean Claire Forbes*
>
> *Claire Forbes, EdD, RN, dean, School of Nursing, Alpha University*
>
> *George Martin, PhD, head, department of English, Ethan Allen College*
>
> *Lesley Prince, DSc, professor, division of social sciences, Alpha University*

Never address an individual as Dr. Claire Forbes, EdD. "Doctor" or "Dr." applies to earned degrees, but its use before a name is commonly identified with medical doctors. Take care to identify a person's specialty if "Doctor" applies to other than a medical doctor.

> *Dr. Janet Van Franken, a registered nurse, writes . . .*
> *Janet Van Franken, DSc, RN* (preferred)

b. *professional titles.*

1. RN (Registered Nurse). Use after the surname except when other titles acknowledge the person as a registered nurse.

2. certification designation (c). The certification symbol (c) appears after the academic degree. In recognizing certified nurses, eliminate the use of RN when the individual's degree is above the baccalaureate.

Sue Shekleton, DNSc, CNM (certified nurse‑midwife)

Jane Monroe, MA, CCRN (certified critical care nurse)

3. FAAN (Fellow of the American Academy of Nursing). Place FAAN at the end of a person's complete title. It is unnecessary to put "RN" after the person's name: all members of the AAN are registered nurses. At the same time, if the audience does not associate FAAN with an RN, then include the latter title.

Margaret A. Lamberson, EdD, FAAN

c. *titles in health care agencies or organizations.* Lowercase except the name of a hospital, health agency, or organization.

Maybelle Crane, MA, CRNA, educational consultant, American Association of Nurse Anesthetists, Park Ridge, IL

Amy Bottoms, MS, FAAN, clinical specialist in psychiatric nursing, Back Bay Mental Health Center, Boston

Martin Johns, MS, assistant director, department of fiscal affairs, Johnson Memorial Medical Center, San Francisco

accept, except. Accept, a verb, means "to receive." Except, a preposition or conjunction, means "other than" or "but for."

As Pearl was about to accept the beautiful bouquet, the embarrassed ballerina suddenly sneezed.

The actor's performance pleased everyone except the impatient understudy.

Also use except as a verb to mean "to leave out."

She was excepted from the new policy.

accreditation/approval. Not synonymous. State board approval is required to operate a school of nursing. Voluntary accreditation is desirable in ensuring high standards.

acts, amendments, bills, laws.   Capitalize acts and laws when refer-ring to their full title or the title by which they are commonly known, such as the *Ohio Nursing Practice Act.* Use lowercase if the act appears alone or in a general explanation.

> *The nursing practice act was one of many such examples.*

Lowercase the names of bills and amendments except when identified with the name of a sponsor, which is capitalized: *the Bradley bill.*

advanced nursing practice.   A term indicating nursing preparation at the master's degree and higher level. Generally refers to nurse practitioners, nurse anesthetists, nurse midwives, and clinical nurse specialists.

adverbs.   Avoid the practice of creating adverbs by adding "ly" to an adjective and then combining it with a weak verb.

> Poor: *To discuss meaningfully*
> Improved: *To enlighten/to persuade/to explain*
>
> Poor: *To think conceptually*
> Improved: *To generate an idea/to conceive an idea*

Put adverbs normally between the elements of a compound verb.

> *We should clearly place more importance on the issue of ethical behavior.*

Do not split an infinitive with an adverb except when the construction appears awkward.

> Awkward: *To place carefully, to alert immediately*
> Improved: *To carefully place, to immediately alert*

adverse, averse. Adverse means "opposed to or unfavorable to"; averse means "unwilling to or reluctant to."

> *The committee's adverse remarks distressed the chairperson.*
> *He was averse to undertaking the treatment.*

advice, advise. Use advice as a noun, advise as a verb.

> *Hillary Marks gave her student valuable advice on career opportunities.*
> *The therapist advised her of the procedure's limitations.*

adviser, advisor. Use either, but be consistent within the same work.

affect, effect. As verbs, affect means "to influence or change"; effect means "to accomplish or cause."

> *"Yo-yo" dieting can severely affect your health.*
> *Good nutrition and an active life-style will effect a better sense of well-being.*

The noun, effect, means "result." The noun, affect, is a term reserved for use in psychological works.

> *One effect of IV drug use is the risk of getting AIDS.*

agenda. Singular. The plural, agendas, is rarely used.

> *No one knew the hidden agenda until the meeting concluded.*

ages. Give the ages of people in numerals, such as *the 5-month-old boy, Margaret Smith, 43 years old.*
  Spell out the ages of inanimate objects or things nine and below, and use figures above nine unless they are round numbers.

The one-hundred-year-old facility, the five-year-old record.

An exception is when both categories appear in a sentence or paragraph discussion.

The one-hundred-year-old institute's twelve branches needed repair.

aggravate, annoy. Not interchangeable. Aggravate means "to make worse, more severe" and annoy is "to disturb or irritate."

Mr. Foote aggravated his back problem by lifting the computer.

Don't annoy the patient with too many questions.

aid, aide. As a verb, aid means "to assist," as a noun, "assistance." Aide, a noun, means "an assistant."

Professor Smart aided her students in resolving the issue.

The students appreciated Professor Smart's aid.

The aide performed her tasks well.

-al. Follow the practice of dropping the terminal al unless it changes the meaning.

Tanya's expertise was in the oncologic (not oncological) field.

When Lincoln delivered the Gettysburg Address, it was an historic (not historical) event.

all ready, already. Used as a pronoun or adjective, all ready means "entirely prepared." Use already, an adverb, to mean "so soon" or "previously."

They were all ready to leave, but the discharge clerk kept them waiting.

The operation was already delayed two hours.

allude, elude. Allude means "to make indirect reference"; elude means "to avoid or escape."

Explaining the new procedure, Roseanne alluded to a change in staffing.
Tom skillfully eluded the instructor's demands.

a lot. Always written as two words meaning "much" or "many." Alot is not a word.

The social worker spent a lot of time contacting agencies.

alumnus, alumni/alumna, alumnae. An alumnus (alumni *pl*) is "a man who has attended or graduated from an institute of higher learning."
An alumna (alumnae *pl*) is the similar reference for a woman. Use alumni to refer to a group of men and women.

A.M., P.M./a.m., p.m. Upper or lowercase, with or without periods, but be consistent. Avoid redundancy such as *10:30 A.M. yesterday morning.* Often printed as small capitals: A.M. 6:00 A.M. is preferable to 6 A.M.

Surgery was scheduled for 8:00 A.M. (Not eight in the A.M.)

among, between. Between applies to two people or things, and among to more than two: *between you and me, among the children.*

ampersand (&). Symbol for "and." Use only in company names and abbreviations, such as *AT&T, Smith & Wesson,* but not in formal writing.

and etc. Because etc. means "and all the rest," the and in and etc. is unnecessary. Suggest substituting "and so on." See Latin derivatives.

and/or.   Used primarily in legal and business writing. Avoid usage in professional writing.

anxious, eager.   Anxious usually means "nervous" or "worried" and describes negative feelings. Eager means "enthusiastically anticipating," describing positive feelings.

> *He was anxious about his medical report.*
> *They were anxious about the imminent birth of Murphy's baby.*
> *She was eager to sign the contract for her first book.*

anyplace.   Avoid this informal expression meaning "anywhere."

apostrophe.   Apostrophes are used to:

- Form the possessive of nouns not ending in s.

  the school's dean, the patient's prescription

- Form the possessive of plural nouns ending in s. Use the apostrophe only.

  nurses' notes, doctors' rounds

- Form the possessive of singular nouns ending in s or s sounds. Use either the apostrophe alone or 's.

  Burns' poetry   Burns's poetry

An exception is the omission of the apostrophe in the proper names of most state and district nurses' associations. This is consistent with the style of the American Nurses Association, as in the *Colorado Nurses Association.*

- Form plurals of letters. Use 's if needed for clarity.

  13 i's   ABCs   CEOs   RNs

- Indicate the omission of one or more letters or figures.

  won't   *the 'gator*   *'93*

- Form the plural of numerals. The trend is to omit the apostrophe, but be consistent.

  1950's (1950s)   *size 10s*   *the 60s*

appraise, apprize, apprise.   Use appraise or apprize to mean "to evaluate"; use apprise for "to inform."

> *The autograph expert appraised the Nightingale letters but did not disclose their value.*
>
> *They apprised the tour leader of the hazardous driving conditions.*

apt, likely, liable.   These three adjectives have subtle differences. Apt means "well adapted," likely means "probably, believable," and liable means "legally obligated, responsible."

> *He made an apt choice.*
>
> *It was a likely story.*
>
> *She admitted that she was liable for her actions.*

armed services, armed forces.   Lowercase unless using the proper name of a specific branch of the military, such as *US Army Nurse Corps*.

as, because, since.   These three conjunctions have slight differences. Use as to convey a specific time instead of while or when. Because and since are interchangeable, showing cause and effect.

> *As the nurse prepared his medication, the patient watched her carefully.*
>
> *Because (since) the student's finances were limited, he bought used textbooks.*

as, like.   A conjunction or preposition, as means "similar" or "similarly to." *Like* is a preposition only.

> *The students used the same equipment on one unit as they did earlier in the classroom.*
>
> *You can get your degree as I did.*
>
> *If he dresses like a physician, people may think he is one.*
>
> *You can go to a university like the one suggested by your counselor.*

assistance, assistants.   Use assistance to mean "support or help," assistants to mean "helpers."

> *Her client's assistance with the test hastened the results.*
>
> *He had openings for two assistants on the project.*

assistant, associate.   Use assistant for a "helper," associate for a "fellow worker" or "partner."

> *My assistant will show you the way.*
>
> *My associate will prepare a draft of the budget.*

In academia, an associate professor ranks below a full professor but above an assistant professor. Never abbreviate either term. Capitalize only when part of a formal title before a name.

> *Assistant Dean Margaret Clinton*

associate of arts, associate of science.   Always use the full title when referring to the degree, usually earned from a junior or community college. ADN commonly refers to an associate degree in nursing.

association.   Capitalize the word when part of an organization's name, as in *American Association of Colleges of Nursing.* Otherwise, lowercase it.

assure, ensure, insure.   All verbs. Assure means "to promise" and refers to persons. Ensure and insure mean "to make certain," but the latter is preferred in legal and financial writing and usually implies formal protective measures.

> *I can assure you that the protocol will be followed.*
> *Her hospitalization ensured proper care.*
> *It is difficult to insure yourself against some natural disasters.*

at large.   Hyphenate only when used as an adjective.

> *She was elected as a delegate at large.*
> *The delegate-at-large elections were held Saturday.*

author.   In the narrative of an article that has a byline, it is more acceptable to use a pronoun to express the author's point of view than to write "the author believes."

> *In my view, . . .* rather than *In this author's view . . . .*
> *I (We) believe . . .* rather than *The author believes . . . .*

Avoid using "to author" as a transitive verb.

> Poor: *Jennifer Penn authored an excellent article on managed care.*
> Improved: *Jennifer Penn was the author of an excellent article on managed care.*

avant-garde.   Always hyphenate.

awful, awfully.   Avoid in formal writing. Substitute a word that closely matches the intended meaning.

> Poor: *Ms. Sanger had an awful delivery.*
> Improved: *Ms. Sanger had a difficult delivery.*

a while, awhile.   Use awhile, an adverb, as one word. Use a while (two words), a noun phrase, after a preposition.

> *The dean decided to wait awhile for the evaluations.*
> *I will complete my introductory courses in a while.*

B

baby girl (or *boy*).   A redundant phrase as in *She delivered a baby girl.* No one is born fully grown.

> *She delivered a six-pound girl.*
> *She delivered a six-pound daughter.*

baccalaureate.   Means "bachelor's degree." The term baccalaureate degree is redundant, although commonly used in education.

> *He earned his baccalaureate with honors.*

bachelor of arts, bachelor of science.   Lower case. Use BA or BS or bachelor's degree. BSN is the abbreviation for a bachelor of science degree in nursing. Always use an apostrophe in bachelor's or master's degree. It is acceptable to say bachelor's without the word degree.

back of, in back of.   Behind is a more acceptable choice.

> *He was behind the podium when the president approached the dais.*

bad, badly.   Bad is an adjective, badly an adverb.

> *He did a bad job on the report.*
> *He did badly on the entrance examination.*

because of, due to.   Use because of, a preposition, to mean "by reason of" or "on account of." Due to is unacceptable as a preposition meaning "because of." In formal writing, use <u>due to</u> only after a form of the verb "to be."

Her irritable behavior was due to a lack of sleep.
Because of (not due to) the patient's high fever, the surgery was postponed.

<u>before, prior to.</u>   <u>Prior to</u> is used most frequently in a legal sense; <u>before</u> is used in almost all other cases.

Prior to rendering an opinion, Judge Eastwood requested a psychiatric evaluation of the felon.
Before starting an infusion, the nurse checked her patient's oral intake.

<u>beside, besides.</u>   A preposition, <u>beside</u> means "next to." An adverb, <u>besides</u> means "in addition to."

Her colleagues stood beside her during the award ceremony.

Besides Ms. Hill, other people shared the organization's convictions.

<u>Besides</u> can be a preposition meaning "in addition to" or "except."

There was no one in the OR suite besides the surgeon, the nurse, and the technician.

<u>biannual, semiannual, biennial.</u>   <u>Biannual</u> and <u>semiannual</u> are synonymous terms meaning twice a year; <u>biennial</u> means every two years.

He recommended a biannual checkup.
ANA and NLN have biennial conventions.

<u>bimonthly, semimonthly.</u>   <u>Bimonthly</u> means "every two months," <u>semimonthly</u> is "twice a month." To avoid confusion, use <u>every two months</u> or <u>twice a month.</u>

black.   Lowercase: *black Americans, the black experience.* See Minority.

blame on.   Avoid this term.

> Poor: *His hospitalization was blamed on his forgetting to take the medicine.*
> Improved: *His forgetfulness to take the medicine was blamed for his hospitalization.*

Because the hospitalization is not the target of the blame, a better form would be:

> *The hospitalization was attributed to his forgetting to take the medicine.*

board of directors, board of trustees, governing board.   Always lowercase except when used with the name of the organization.

> *The board of directors voted to suspend debate.*
> *He was elected to the AHA Board of Trustees.*

buzzword.   A word used by members in a particular discipline or profession. Avoid in formal writing.

C

can, may.   Use can to convey "ability" or "capacity" as well as "possibility." Use may to convey "permission."

> *She can run a successful business and still be a good wife and mother.*
> *May I go to the workshop?*

capital, capitol.   Lowercase when referring to capital, the city or town that is the seat of government. Uppercase when capitol refers to a specific national or state building.

The nurses met with their representatives in the state capital.
The nurses lobbied their legislators at the State Capitol.

capitalization.   In general, limit capitalization to proper nouns.
a. *organizations.* Capitalize only when the official name of the entire organization, body, or group is given.

University of Minnesota School of Nursing	*the school of nursing*
the Board of Review for Baccalaureate and Higher Degree Programs	*the board of review*
the NLN Board of Directors	*the board of directors, the board*

Exception: Use *the League* when referring to the National League for Nursing. Refer to a constituent league as *the league.*

b. *titles.* Capitalize only in lists or when the title precedes the name.

Dean Donna Sharpe	*Donna Sharpe, dean of the school*
Executive Director David A. Bean	*David A. Bean, executive director*

c. *courses, workshops.* Capitalize specific courses or workshops. No quotes. Lowercase the names of subjects.

Ethical/Legal Aspects of Nursing	*a course in ethics in nursing*
Chemistry 102	*chemistry*
a conference on Patterns in Specialization: Challenge to the Curriculum	*a conference on specialization in nursing*

caregiver, caretaker.   Use caregiver in lieu of caretaker when referring to a person involved in the health care of an individual.

<u>Caretaker</u> is generally used to describe a person employed to take care of property.

catalog, catalogue.   Catalog is the preferred spelling, but be consistent.

Celsius.   Named after the person who invented the centigrade system. Commonly used in scientific writing: *46 degrees Celsius or 40°C.* Fahrenheit, also named for its inventor, is rarely used.

chair, chairperson.   <u>Chairperson</u> is the preferred alternative to chairman or chairwoman, particularly in academia and government. Use the term <u>chair</u> for either gender. Capitalize only when used as a formal title before a name.

> *Chairperson Marguerite Lopez called the meeting to order.*
>
> *The chair called the meeting to order.*

check up, checkup.   Use <u>check up</u> as a verb, <u>checkup</u> as a noun.

> *Monica's anxiety delayed her checkup.*
>
> *The new pharmacist decided to check up on the narcotics supply.*

cities and states.   Capitalize names of cities and towns. Do not capitalize the word <u>city</u> unless it is part of the official name, such as Kansas City. Otherwise, lowercase, such as *the city of Boston.*

Unless a mailing address is being given, the name of the state should follow the city except in the case of major cities, such as *Atlanta, Boston, Chicago, Denver, Iowa City, Los Angeles, New York,* and so on.

Spell out in full the name of a state when it stands alone, but abbreviate it when it follows the name of a city. Use the U.S. Postal Service abbreviations for state names.

> *Ohio   Columbus, OH   Oregon   Portland, OR*

Spell out the name of a state when it follows the name of a county.

Montgomery County, Pennsylvania
Cook County, Illinois

Do not repeat the name of a state when it is included in the name of an institution or organization.

University of Minnesota, Minneapolis
Arkansas Department of Health, Little Rock

In all but major foreign cities, follow the name of the city with the full name of the country.

Amsterdam   London   Paris   Tokyo   New Delhi
Castlecomer, Ireland   Limoges, France

Enclose the abbreviation of a state in parenthesis when identifying the name of a hospital or health agency.

Coral Gables (FL) Memorial Medical Center

clinical ladder.   In nursing, refers to a system of recognition and reward to nurses meeting special criteria at different levels of practice. Also describes progress of the nurse advancing from one level or step to another.

clinical nurse specialist.   Refers to a registered nurse prepared at the master's degree level or higher in a clinical nursing specialty.

collective noun.   A unit taking singular verbs and pronouns.

The staff performs self-scheduling.
The jury is confined behind closed doors.

colon. Marks the beginning of a phrase or sentence. Also used to introduce an important quote or a series. Capitalize the first word after a colon if a complete sentence follows.

> _His therapy served a purpose: It helped to build up his confidence._
>
> _His therapy could be described this way: effective, timely, and expensive._

comma. Punctuation mark used to separate elements in a series, and generally before a conjunction. Often overused.

> _The top candidates were Joan, Jill, and Jessica._

Avoid the common error of inserting a comma to separate two or more verbs having the same subject.

> Poor: _The nurse took the chart, and recorded the patient's vital signs._
>
> Improved: _The nurse took the chart and recorded the patient's vital signs._

committee, commission. As collective nouns, committee and commission can take singular verbs if considered a singular unit. (See verb agreement.) Capitalize only when part of a proper name. Do not abbreviate.

> _The Pew Health Professions Commission issued a visionary report._
>
> _The committee believes that its recommendations are sound._

company, companies. Capitalize only when part of a proper name, such as _American Journal of Nursing Company._

compare to, with. Use compare to when the sense is "to consider or describe resemblances between unlike things." Use compare with to show similarities or differences between two like things.

The committee compared the woman's report of the incident to a soap opera script.

The nurse activists compared their efforts on the Equal Rights Amendment with Lavinia Dock's work in women's suffrage.

<u>compass points.</u>

a. <u>east</u> *(west,* <u>north,</u> <u>south).</u> Capitalize when referring to a geographic region of the country or part of a proper name. Lowercase when you mean a point on a compass.

He left the South to find his fame and fortune on Broadway.

Proceed west on Route 138 for five miles.

Nursing in the Midwest is quite advanced.

She attended a baccalaureate program on the East Coast.

North Carolina, West Virginia

b. <u>eastern</u> *(*<u>western,</u> <u>northern,</u> <u>southern).</u> Capitalize when referring to a geographic area of the country.

Bill has a Southern accent.

Milly is a Northerner.

Lowercase to designate compass points of a section of a state or city.

western New Hampshire

southern Dallas

It is acceptable, however, to capitalize widely known compass points such as *Southern California* or *Lower East Side of New York.* If in doubt, lower case.

<u>complement, compliment.</u>   Noun or verb. <u>Complement</u> means "that which completes or makes perfect"; a <u>compliment</u> is "an expression of praise."

The support of the family complemented the patient's treatment.

The physical therapist complimented the elderly woman on her progress.

complementary, complimentary. Use complementary to mean "serving as a complement, completing"; use complimentary to mean "given as an act of courtesy" and, in some cases, "free."

The efforts of the health care team showed a complementary relationship.

She received a complimentary book for her efforts.

compose, comprise, consist of, constitute. These commonly misused words have subtle differences:

- compose: "to create or put together."
- comprise: "to contain; to include for all to embrace."
- consist of: "to be made up of."
- constitute: "to make up or form."

The nutritionist composed a 24-hour instruction plan.

Two nurses, a physician, and an administrator comprised the committee.

Seventy percent of the board constitutes a quorum.

His breakfast consisted of cereal, milk, and fruit.

conference, congress, convention. Capitalize when part of a proper noun or as a title of an event. Otherwise, lowercase.

The 1993 NLN Conference on Gerontological Nursing featured outstanding faculty.

The ICN Congress drew thousands of international participants.

APHA held its recent convention in Washington, DC.

Congressman, Congresswoman.   Capitalize only when used with a proper name. Refer to a member of the House as, for example, *Representative Barbara Sparks;* thereafter, refer to the individual as *the congresswoman.*

> *Congressman Trueheart gave a fine address.*
> *Several of the state congressmen rejected his comment.*

connote, denote.   Connote means "to suggest or imply something beyond the explicit meaning." Denote means "to be explicit about the meaning."

> *To some nurses, the concept of graduate education for certification connotes a threat.*
> *To others, certification denotes the appropriate mechanism for fostering higher standards in nursing.*

continual, continuous.   Use continual to mean "repeated often" or "intermittent," and continuous to mean "uninterrupted, without stopping."

> *Her continual habit of forgetting to take the medicine frustrated her family.*
> *The award recognized the association's continuous support of health care reform.*

contrast to, contrast with.   Use contrast to to refer to something that is "opposite," and contrast with to mean "different."

> *Her reaction to the diagnosis was in contrast to her husband's response.*
> *The contrast with her staff's opinion appeared obvious to everyone but the nurse manager.*

council, counsel.   Use council, a noun, to mean "a group of advisers." Use counsel, a verb, to mean "to give advice." As a noun, counsel means "advice given."

The President's Council meets bimonthly.

They counsel recovering alcoholics.

She followed the counsel of the chief financial officer.

credible, creditable, credulous.   Use credible to mean "believable" and creditable to mean "worthy." A credulous person is "gullible."

The report was complicated but appeared credible to the nurse executives.

In substituting for her colleague, Ms. Jones gave a creditable performance.

The credulous student concurred with the instructor's analysis.

criteria, criterion.   Use criteria, the plural of criterion, to mean "standards for judgment."

Of all the criteria for selecting the candidate, character was considered the most important criterion.

current, present.   Synonymous terms meaning "belonging in the present" or "generally accepted."

The past results were low, whereas the current figures showed improvement.

In many cases, use of either word is unnecessary.

Poor: *The current president of Sigma Theta Tau International will speak.*

Improved: *The president of Sigma Theta Tau International will speak.*

currently, presently.   Synonymous adverbs. It is more acceptable, however, to use presently to mean "shortly, soon, or now."

The discharge planner is (currently) unavailable but will be here presently.

curriculum. The preferred plural is curriculums, rather than curricula.

cutoff, cut off. Use the noun cutoff to mean a "termination point." Do not use as an adjective. Cut off, a verb, means "to interrupt or sever."

> *The cutoff for the application is February 1.*
> *The moderator cut off the panelist who spoke too long.*

D

dash. Punctuation mark showing a break in thought in a sentence, or emphasizing an appositive, or setting off parenthetical phrases.

> *In addition to the large group meetings, there were seven smaller breakout sessions—led by trained facilitators—whereby each participant remained with the same group and leader throughout the conference.*

Avoid when a comma will suffice.

> Poor: *These three elements—character, compassion, and credentials—combine to produce a qualified candidate.*
> Improved: *These three elements, character, compassion, and credentials, combine to produce a qualified candidate.*

datum, data. Use data as the plural of datum in formal writing. When the group or quantity is considered a unit, it is acceptable to use data as a collective noun with a singular verb. In lieu of datum, use "fact" or "figure."

> *The data are carefully recorded into the computer.*
> *The data* (a unit) *is valid.*

days of the week.   Always capitalize. Abbreviate in a manuscript only when used in a tabular format.

diagnosis, prognosis.   Diagnosis identifies a disease through examination; prognosis predicts the disease outcome.

dietitian, nutritionist.   A dietitian is a person specializing in the study of nutrition as it relates to health. A nutritionist is an expert in the study of foods in general.

> *The hospital dietitian is responsible for planning patients' meals.*
> *She attributed her weight loss and energy to the nutritionist's teachings.*

different from, different than.   Use different from except when a clause follows, and different than when different from would sound awkward.

> *The protocols this year are different from those followed last year.*
> *It's a different procedure than it was 15 years ago.*

dilemma.   Watch the spelling and meaning of this word. Dilemma isn't just a problem, but one involving a choice between alternatives.

> *The dilemma facing her was either to report the mistake or to respect her best friend's confidence.*

disability.   See Section V, B.

discreet, discrete.   Use discreet to mean "tactful," and discrete for "separate."

> *She offered a discreet comment about the controversy.*
> *They discussed the discrete elements of the plan.*

disease entities. Do not capitalize a disease entity unless used with a proper noun: *cancer, asthma, coronary disease, Bright's disease, Hodgkin's disease, Alzheimer's disease.* Use lowercase for procedures such as *cesarean* (or *cesarian*) *section.*

disinterested, uninterested. Use *disinterested* to mean "unbiased or impartial," *uninterested* for "bored or lacking interest."

> *Most staff nurses were disinterested in the outcome of the dispute.*
> *The technician was uninterested in her explanation of the problem.*

doctorate. A noun synonymous with "doctoral degree." Do not use as an adjective.

> Poor: *Jerry earned his doctorate degree.*
> Improved: *Jerry earned his doctoral degree (or his doctorate).*

documentation. See *referencing.*

domestic violence. Preferred usage to "family abuse."

don't, doesn't. Do not confuse *don't*, the contraction for "do not," and *doesn't*, the contraction for "does not."

dose, dosage. Use *dosage* to mean "a prescribed amount of a therapeutic agent." *Dose*, an abbreviation, is "an agent taken at one time or at stated intervals."

> *The dosage prescribed for Mr. Payne's headache was ineffective.*
> *The primary nurse gave the patient his 10 o'clock dose of pain medication.*

double negatives. Unacceptable.

> Poor: *The unit clerk didn't have nothing to do on her personal day.*

Improved: *The unit clerk didn't have anything to do on her personal day.*

doubt that, doubt whether, doubt if.   Use doubt that to express conviction, doubt whether and doubt if to show uncertainty.

I doubt that she intended to hurt his feelings.
I doubt whether (if) the board understood the ramifications of its decision.

E

each, every.   Use "each" or "every" in place of phrases such as "each and every."

Each of us agreed with the diagnosis.
Every one of the patients was awake and hungry.

When each is used as a pronoun, it takes a singular verb.

Each was well educated for the task at hand.

When each follows a plural subject, the verb agrees with the subject.

The patients each have separate rooms.

editor in chief.   Preferred style is not to hyphenate. Follow, however, the style of the journal or the individual's title as indicated in correspondence.

e.g.   See Latin derivatives.

-elect.   Always hyphenate words formed with -elect, such as *president-elect, chairperson-elect.*

ellipses. (. . .)   These marks appear in threes and fours. Three dots represent words omitted from within or at the beginning of a sentence. Four dots (actually a period linked to three dots) show that words have been omitted at the end of a sentence or that sentences have been omitted from a paragraph.

eminent, imminent.   Use eminent to mean "distinguished," imminent to mean "something about to occur."

> *The eminent scientist keynoted the convention.*
> *The beginning of the convention processional was imminent.*

end run, end-run.   Both the noun, end run, and the transitive verb, end-run, are informal terms and have no place in professional writing.

especially, particularly, specially.   Especially and particularly are interchangeable. Specially means "for a specific reason."

> *I especially (particularly) enjoy the fringe benefits of my job.*
> *The conference was specially designed for health professionals.*

essential clauses.   Clauses are "essential" if they restrict the meaning. No commas.

> *Undergraduate students who have a 3.5 average are eligible for the dean's list.*
> *Deadlines that are not met will age editors early.*

et al.   See Latin derivatives.

et cetera.   See Latin derivatives.

everyone, everybody.   Synonyms that take a singular verb.

> *Everybody respects Emily, and everyone supported her promotion to nurse manager.*

ex-.   In formal writing, former is preferred to use of ex-.

The decline in cigarette smoking among American adults has resulted in many healthier former smokers.

exclamation (!).   Reserve this punctuation mark for true exclamations or commands. Do not use merely to emphasize a simple statement.

It was an exciting conference.
What an exciting conference!

expired.   Use died rather than expired or passed away.

Poor: *Mr. Welles collapsed on the steps and expired within minutes.*
Improved: *Mr. Welles collapsed on the steps and died within minutes.*

explicit, implicit.   Use explicit to mean "clearly defined," implicit to mean "implied" or "understood."

We have an implicit understanding that the children may not watch movies containing explicit sex.

F

farther, further.   Use farther, an adverb, to show physical space; use further, an adjective or adverb, to indicate "for an additional time" or "in a greater amount," or in relation to abstract ideas.

The ambulance was farther from the hospital than she had thought.
She did not wish to discuss the issue further.
Needing further consultation, the attending physician called in his colleagues.

There isn't anything further from the truth.

Use <u>further</u>, a verb, to mean "to advance."

She needed funds to further her education.

<u>federal</u>.   Capitalize for corporate or governmental bodies that use the word as part of their formal names: *the Federal Trade Commission, Federal Express.* More common practice is lowercase when used as an adjective synonymous with the United States, such as *federal judge, federal agents, federal grants,* and so on.

<u>feminist</u>.   Describes a person whose beliefs and behavior are based on social, economic, and political equality of the sexes. Can be applied to a person of either sex.

<u>fewer, less</u>.   Use <u>fewer</u>, a plural noun, when referring to a number or group of individual persons or items. <u>Less</u>, a singular noun, refers to quantities of abstract or unnumbered entities. Both words imply comparison: "fewer than," "less than."

> *Medical schools received fewer applications from men last year.*
> *The medical center received less criticism than its board of directors had expected.*

<u>figurative language</u>.   Refers to words used non-literally. The basis of figurative language is comparison or association of two ordinarily separate things or ideas. Become familiar with the following common figures of speech:

a. <u>*metaphor*</u>.   An implied non-literal comparison. Avoid using "like" or "as," or other words implying a comparison. Examples of metaphors are:

> *Why then **the world's mine oyster** . . . .* ("The Merry Wives of Windsor," William Shakespeare)
> *This is **the porcelain clay of humankind**.* ("Don Sebastian," John Dryden)

. . . leave behind us **footprints on the sands of time.**
("Psalm of Life," Henry Wadsworth Longfellow)

Avoid trite metaphors such as *cradle of the deep* or *captain of my soul.*

b. *mixed metaphors.* Two or more dissimilar images presented in rapid succession. Avoid them.

The medical center fiscally solved **a sea of problems** *when unexpected funding propelled it into* **the lap of luxury.**

c. *simile.* A non-literal comparison of two things dissimilar in most respects but similar to each other. Usually introduced by "like" or "as." Use sparingly if at all.

When he defected from the Party, he acted **like a bird out of a cage.**

Avoid trite similes such as *soft as a kitten, happy as a lark, pretty as a picture, hard as nails,* and *nutty as a fruitcake* (slang).

figuratively, literally.   Use figuratively to mean "involving a figure of speech or emblematic." It implies a nonfactual statement. Literally means "actually."

Observing her first operation, the young student literally fainted at the open operating sight.
The evaluations committee described her proposal figuratively as a fairy tale.

finalize.   Avoid in formal writing. Considered corporate and bureaucratic jargon. See ize.

first, firstly.   First, second, and so on are preferred although firstly, secondly, and so on are grammatically correct. Be consistent in the form used.

following, after.   An adjective, following means "coming next in order." After, a preposition, means "behind in place or sequence."

> *Watch for the following protocol.*
> *She spoke after the award luncheon.* (Never use *following the luncheon.*)

follow-through, follow-up.   Follow-up is also an adjective. Both can be used as verbs without hyphens.

footnotes.   See referencing.

foreword, forward.   Use the noun foreword for an introductory section of a book. As a verb, forward means "to advance"; as an adjective, it means "ahead" or "front."

> *Ms. Joslin wrote an excellent foreword to the text on diabetes education.*
> *Please move forward or we will miss the speaker.*
> *The forward pass was the chief weapon in the quarterback's arsenal.*

formally, formerly.   Use formally to mean "in a formal manner" and formerly to mean "previously."

> *The chairperson formally convened the curriculum committee.*
> *She practiced formerly in a community health agency in Atlanta.*

former, latter.   An adjective, former means "something that occurred earlier in time, or that which came before." As a noun, it means "the first of two items." Use latter to refer to the second of a pair.

> *Her former employer was his former wife.*
> *When Jay had to choose between a salad and soup, he selected the former.*

Johnny and Ed are being interviewed, but the latter may drop out of the running.

full-time, full time/part-time, part time.   Hyphenate as an adjective (compound modifier) but not as a noun or adverb.

She has a full-time job.
She works full time.

fulsome.   Adjective meaning "offensively lavish." Not synonymous with "profuse." The use of the term "fulsome praise" (to mean abundant) is ambiguous and might cause confusion. A word such as "full" or "abundant" leaves no doubt of the meaning.

G

gentleman, gentlemen.   Man or men is preferred.

geriatric nursing, gerontological nursing.   Geriatric nursing literally means "nursing care of the aged." Gerontological nursing means "nursing care of the aged with emphasis on health, rather than on illness." (Historical note: In 1976, the ANA Division on Geriatric Nursing Practice became the ANA Division on Gerontological Nursing Practice, to reflect a focus on health.)
    Despite the different shades of meaning, the terms are often used interchangeably as in geriatric nurse practitioner (or specialist) and gerontological nurse practitioner (or specialist).

geriatrics, gerontology.   Not interchangeable. Geriatrics is "the study of diseases of the aged." Gerontology is "the study of normal aging."

gerunds.   See verbals.

girl.   Do not use in references to a woman or a young woman. College student is preferable to college girl.

good, well.   Good, an adjective, describes someone or something; well, an adverb, describes an action. When used with verbs such as "look," "to be," or "feel," well refers to a state of health.

> *She is a good physician, but a difficult patient.*
> *The staff on 2-Miller work well together.*
> *The project is going well.*
> *I feel well.*
> *She looks well after her illness.*

got, gotten.   As a past participle of get, got (also the simple past tense of get) is preferred to gotten, the colloquial past participle of get.

> *She finally got the message.* (past)
> *He didn't mean to volunteer, but he got caught up in the enthusiasm of the event.*

government.   Lowercase. Never abbreviate.

> *the federal government, the state government, the U.S. government*

governmental bodies.   Use full names. Capitalize the full proper name of governmental agencies, departments, and offices: *U.S. Department of Health and Human Services.* Lowercase further mention of the name, such as *the department.*

graduate, graduated.   Always use from with the verb graduate.

> Poor: *She graduated Teachers College, Columbia University.*
> Improved: *She graduated from Teachers College, Columbia University.*

grandfather/grandmother clause.   Term meaning "a clause creating an exemption based on circumstances previously existing." To avoid sexism, contemporary usage is <u>grandperson clause</u> or <u>grand-persoing</u> in lieu of <u>grandfathering</u> or <u>grandmothering.</u>

grassroots.   One word. Although a plural noun, <u>grassroots</u> often modifies another noun, such as *grassroots member, grassroots movement.*

> *The message from the grassroots favored action on a national health insurance plan.*

When used as a subject, <u>grassroots</u> uses either a singular or plural verb.

> *The grassroots is (are) concerned about the economy.*

<u>*ground rules.*</u>   Omit "ground" unless referring to sports.

H

health care.   Two words, but observe exceptions in formal names such as *The Joint Commission on Accreditation of Healthcare Agencies.* Hyphenate sparingly when used as an adjective.

> *The health care industry is flourishing.*
> *The nurses provide home health care.*

healthful, healthy.   Use <u>healthful</u> to mean "conducive to good health" and <u>healthy</u> to mean "possessing good health."

> *In addition to being healthy, the nutritionist recommended healthful foods to her clients.*

<u>*help, help but.*</u>   Avoid the phrase "help but."

> Poor: *He couldn't help but admire her commitment.*
> Improved: *He couldn't help admiring her commitment.*

historic, historical.   An historic event is one that stands out in history. An historical event refers to any past occurrence.

> *The NLN's 100th anniversary, observed in Boston, was an historic event.*
>
> *At the convention, the organization displayed many historical materials.*

home care.   Two words. Hyphenate sparingly when used as an adjective.

homosexual, lesbian.   Use these terms rather than "gay" in formal writing.

hopefully.   An adverb, hopefully means "with hope." Avoid using hopefully in formal writing when the meaning is "it is hoped."

> *It is hoped that writers will strive to master the use of the word "hopefully."*

however.   According to most grammarians, however, an adverb, should not begin a sentence.

> Poor: *The film received a favorable review. However, it did not meet the expectations of the audience.*
>
> Improved: *The film received a favorable review. It did not, however, meet the expectations of the audience.*

To avoid such binds, rework the sentence as follows:

> *Although the film received a favorable review, it did not meet the audience's expectations.*

hyphen.   Two principles: Never divide words of one syllable and hyphenate only between syllables.
    Use a hyphen to avoid ambiguity when forming a single idea from two or more words.

The administrator will speak to small-business men.

He re-covered the wound with a sterile dressing.

Do not hyphenate an adverb ending in l̲y̲ and a participle. Examples are: *easily remembered dosages, slowly moving car.*

Use hyphens between two or more modifiers that express a single thought, except in the above-mentioned example.

a full-time employee

300-bed hospital

anxiety-provoking situation

Hyphens are used when a word breaks at the end of a line of print. Avoid more than two successive lines that end with hyphens. Consult a dictionary for correct word breaks.

Ms. Henderson responded in a professional manner to the allegation.

Her recent article presented timely information.

I̲

I. Use of the pronoun "I" in a manuscript can be effective if it is not overdone. Check the style of the target publication. Former United Press International editor Roger Tatarian said: "There should be enough of it [I] to give the flavor of the letter to the folks at home, but not so much as to make the writer hog the center of the stage."

i̲d̲iom. An expression unique to a specific profession, group of people or region of the country. As slang or near slang, idioms are often peculiar grammatically and cannot be understood merely from the meaning of their elements, such as *get the upper hand, keep tabs on, gone to the dogs, strike a bargain.* Idioms are not recommended for professional writing.

impact.   A noun or verb indicating "forceful contact."

The rock impacted the car and forced the driver to lose control.

Do not use impact to mean "having an effect on."

Poor: *The decision impacted the association.*
Improved: *The decision had an impact on the association.*

imply, infer.   Not synonymous. Imply means "to suggest or to hint"; infer means "to conclude from evidence, to draw a conclusion." A speaker implies something, whereas a listener infers something from a speaker.

The lab report implies serious problems ahead.
The results of the lab test led us to infer serious problems ahead.

in, into.   Use in to indicate a state or position. Into describes a movement to an interior location or condition.

He was suffering in his anguish.
Throw the recyclables into the bin!

incredible, incredulous.   Use incredible to mean "unbelievable," incredulous to mean "skeptical."

His explanation was incredible.
The administrator gave him an incredulous stare.

infinitive, split infinitive.   See adverbs, verbals.

ingenious, ingenuous, disingenuous.   A confusing trio of similar-sounding words. Use ingenious to mean "displaying ingenuity, springing from an imaginative mind," ingenuous to mean "innocent, lacking sophistication," and disingenuous to mean "not straightforward, crafty."

The staff praised her ingenious solution to the problem.
The ingenuous newcomer captivated her classmates.
His disingenuous comments aroused suspicion.

input. As a noun and verb, <u>input</u> is a technical term to describe information entered into a computer or word processing system. Input, the noun, also means an "amount entered to achieve an output," such as *an input of fuel.*

The statistician used her data as input for the computer.
She spent hours inputting the information into the new database.

In professional writing, avoid <u>input</u> as a noun meaning "general information" when "information" or "data" will suffice.

Poor: *She received valuable input for her report.*
Improved: *She received valuable information (or data) for her report.*

introductory expressions. Set off by commas, such expressions include <u>for example</u>, <u>namely</u>, <u>such as</u>, and <u>that is</u>. If the break in continuity is minor, no comma is necessary. Use a semicolon or a dash for a major break.

The computer output, for example, was a daily printout on each patient.
The instructor postponed the assignment, namely the two essays.

in-service. Never convert the adjective <u>in-service</u> to a noun or verb. Hyphenate.

Poor: *We will in-service the new staff next week.*
Improved: *We will begin the in-service program for staff next week.*

italics.   Italicize or underline names of books, newspapers, and magazines. Use quotation marks around the names of chapters, articles, lecture or speech titles, television programs, movies, plays, poems, or songs.

> *Nursing and Health Care has a wide distribution.*
> *Most academics follow The Chronical of Higher Education.*
> *The children repeatedly asked to watch the tape of "Snow White and the Seven Dwarfs."*

it's, its.   It's is a contraction meaning "it is." Its is the possessive form of the pronoun "it."

> *It's the unit's decision to determine its staff scheduling.*

ize.   The suffix ize is a convenient way to turn nouns into verbs, as in jeopardize and computerize. Many verbs formed in this manner are bureaucratic and corporate jargon such as *prioritize, operationalize, privatize, accessorize,* and *finalize.* Avoid in professional writing.

J

jargon.   A special language of a trade, profession, class, fellowship, or region of the country. Avoid "jargonitis" such as:

> *Give him some TLC.*
> *Ground the patient.*
> *Check the meds.*

Idioms fall within this category.

K

kids.   Skip such colloquial expressions. Substitute children.

kind, kinds. Use with the demonstrative pronouns *this*, *that* and *these*, *those*: *this kind, that kind; these kinds, those kinds.*

know-how. A trite expression; avoid it in formal writing.

kudos. Takes a singular verb. Never use "kudo."

L

lady, woman. Use woman, not lady, in professional writing.

last, past. Use last to mean "most recent," past to mean "an elapsed time or location."

> *Margo Preston was elected chairperson at the group's last convention.*
>
> *The smell of cotton candy evoked an image of summers past.*

Latin derivatives. Avoid in professional writing. Spell out the English translation. The most common examples are:

- e.g. = *exempli gratia* = for example. Use only if the illustration being offered is one of several possible examples.
- et al. = *and other people* (acceptable in citations only).
- etc. = et cetera = *and other things* (literal). *And so on* is preferable.
- i.e. = *id est* = that is. Used to interpret a previous statement (in which case you probably should have said it more clearly the first time) or to present an exhaustive list of examples.
- viz. = *videlicet* = namely.

lay, lie. Lay means to place, to put in a particular position. It always takes a direct object. Laid is the form for the past tense and past participle. Laying is the present participle.

She laid the dressing on the sterile area.
She is laying the report on the table.
Please lay your head on my shoulder.

Lie means "a state of reclining" and does not take a direct object. Past tense is lay, past participle is lain, and present participle is lying. Lie also means "make an untrue statement."

He was terminated from the project because he lied consistently.
The patient lies quietly in her bed.
He had lain for a long time on the examining table.
She is lying on the unaffected side.
The report lay on the table.

lead, led. As a verb, lead means "to take or conduct." Led is the past tense of lead.

The aide agreed to lead the family into the waiting room.
She led the people through the new wing.

leave, let. Interchangeable only when followed by alone. Otherwise, let means "to allow" and leave "to depart."

Leave (let) the report alone.
Let the patient see the report.

legislative titles. Capitalize titles used with proper names. Abbreviations, such as Rep., Reps., Sen., and Sens., are acceptable before one or more names in regular text.

Sen. Daniel P. Moynihan (D-NY) supported the higher education bill.
The New York senator said he believed the legislation was necessary to achieve the nation's long-term goals.

loath, loathe.   An adjective, <u>loath</u> means "unwilling or reluctant." A verb, <u>loathe</u> means "to detest greatly."

> *He was loath to admit his misjudgment of the employee.*
> *She loathed her job.*

long-term.   Hyphenate as an adjective, but not as a noun or adverb.

> *The health care team agreed on long-term goals involving staff in shared governance.*
> *It is important to consider the results over the long term.*

loose, lose.   An adjective, <u>loose</u> means "free" or "unattached." A verb, <u>lose</u> means "to part with unintentionally."

> *The dressing was loose again.*
> *Don't lose the opportunity to submit your abstract.*

M

majority, plurality.   Use <u>majority</u> to mean "more than half of an amount" and <u>plurality</u> for "greater" or "more than the next highest number." When majority or plurality stands alone, use a singular verb. If a plural word follows <u>majority of</u> or <u>plurality of</u>, use either a singular or plural verb, depending on the meaning of the sentence.

> *The majority elects.*
> *The majority of nurses disagree with the decision.*
> *She won by a narrow plurality.*
> *His plurality was 10,000 votes.*

male nurse.   When necessary to identify a nurse by gender, the appropriate usage is <u>male nurse</u>, not man nurse. Avoid using <u>man</u> as an adjective.

master of arts, master of science.   Lowercase. Abbreviations such as MA, MS, MPH, EdM, and MBA are acceptable in professional writing. No periods are necessary, but be consistent in usage. Always use an apostrophe for "master's degree" and "master's degree program."

> *He expects to earn his master's degree in 1994.*
>
> *She graduated from the master's degree program in psychology.*

media.   Avoid the use of media to mean "a type of mass communication." Terms such as *the press, journalism, newspapers,* and *electronic press* are preferable. Media is the plural of medium.

medical-surgical.   Hyphenate rather than use a slash as in medical/surgical nursing, except when a proper name indicates otherwise.

memorandum.   Use memorandums as the preferred plural, rather than memoranda.

metaphor.   See figurative language.

methodology, method.   Use method to mean the plans or procedures to accomplish a goal, and methodology to mean "principles referring to theoretical analysis."

> *He found a satisfactory method to organize his work.*
>
> *The committee rejected her research because of faulty methodology.*

minority.   Defined as an ethnic, religious, political, national, or other group regarded as different from the larger group of which it is a part. When referring to an ethnic, religious, political, national, or other group, the trend is to substitute people of color rather than the term minority.

> Poor: *Ruth was the first minority person to serve as president.*
>
> Improved: *Ruth was the first person of color to serve as president.*

modifiers. Words, phrases, or clauses in a sentence that limit or explain something. Proper placement is important to avoid confusion.

   a. *dangling modifiers.*

   Poor: *Weighing the options carefully, a decision was made.*
   Improved: *Weighing the options carefully, they decided . . . .*

   b. *misplaced modifiers.*

   Poor: *The patient gave the nurse an incomplete history because of her anxiety.* (Is it the patient's anxiety or the nurse's?)
   Improved: *Because of her anxiety, the patient gave the nurse an incomplete history.*

money, monies. Use money a collective noun and avoid the plural monies.

months. Always capitalize. Do not separate a month and year with a comma when there is no specific date. Do not abbreviate in professional writing.

   He was born in January 1952.
   He was born on January 28, 1952.

When using months in tabular form, use three-letter forms without a period.

   Jan, Feb, Mar, Apr, May, Jun, Jul, Aug, Sep, Oct, Nov, Dec

more important, more importantly. Whenever possible, rephrase a sentence to avoid the use of more importantly (adverb) or more important (adjective).

   Poor: *Her report was more important than mine; more importantly, she received greater visibility.*

Improved: *Her report was more timely than mine. What's more, she received greater visibility.*

Mr., Mrs., Ms., Messrs.   Most publications omit these titles after giving the full name. Although it is suggested to use only the surname, follow the preferred style of the target journal. In situations where the person has an earned doctoral degree, the use of Dr. is optional.

Hope Smith, PhD, and Rachel Bernini, MSN, were assigned to the case. Both Smith and Bernini agreed that it was a challenging task.

N

nationalities and races.   Capitalize the proper names of nationalities, people, races, and tribes, such as: *African-American, American, Arab, Asian, Caucasian, Cherokee, Chinese, Hispanic, Jewish, and Native American.* See minority.

nauseous, nauseated.   An adjective, nauseous means "causes nausea." A verb, nauseated means "to suffer from nausea."

She complained about the nauseous taste of the new medication. The new medicine nauseated her.

necessitate, require.   Use necessitate, a transitive verb, to imply unavoidability. Use require to mean "to need or to have need for."

The emergency operation necessitated a change in the staff's schedule.
His injuries required immediate surgical intervention.

none.   Means "no one, not one, or not any." Singular or plural, depending on meaning.

Of all the concerns, none is more pressing than the credentialing quagmire. (singular)

None of the charges against her is serious. (singular)

Almost none of the professors were interviewed by the dean. (plural)

None but Debbie's greatest admirers support her election. (plural)

<u>not only, but also</u>.   Avoid misplacement of this pair.

Poor: *It would not only be inappropriate, but also untimely.*

Improved: *It would be not only inappropriate, but also untimely.*

The word "also" may be omitted if it does not impair the balance of the sentence.

It would be not only inappropriate, but untimely as well.

<u>numerals</u>.   Write out cardinal and ordinal numerals from one to ten; use numerals for numbers above ten.

Abe walked six miles to the schoolhouse.

By the time he began his practice, Charlton had undergone more than 12 years of preparation.

Anna was in the fifth grade when she decided to become a teacher.

Avoid using numerals at the beginning of a sentence.

Poor: *Fifteen hundred nurse practitioners attended the workshop on women's health.*

Improved: *The workshop on women's health drew 1500 nurse practitioners.*

In money amounts of more than a million, use the currency sign and spell out million, billion, and so on: *$2 million, $28.5 billion.* Use round numbers when appropriate.

Common fractions should be spelled out, as in *half the members, a three-fourths majority.* Use numerals for mixed fractions as in *2½ hours.*

Avoid adding n̲d̲, t̲h̲, s̲t̲ to dates.

Poor: *June 2nd, March 5th, May 1st, 1993.*
Improved: *June 2, March 5, May 1, 1993.*

nurse executive.   Term generally applied to the nurse in the top management position and to some in middle management positions.

nurse manager.   A nurse heading a patient care unit, responsible and accountable for the 24-hour management of that unit.

nurse practitioner.   Refers to a registered nurse prepared at the master's degree level or higher, who provides primary health care.

nursing.   Generally, lowercase.

Flo decided on a career in nursing.

O

of.   Avoid using o̲f̲ with adjectives or adverbs, such as h̲o̲w̲ and t̲o̲o̲.

Poor: *How long of a recovery do you anticipate?*
      It's too complicated of a task to complete in one day.
Improved: *How long a recovery do you anticipate?*
         It's too complicated a task to complete in one day.

office.   Capitalize only when used as part of an agency's or institution's formal name. Lowercase all other uses.

> *The Oval Office of the President*
> *The instructor's office*

OK, OK'd, okay, ok'ing.   Use only for informal speech and writing.

on one hand, on the other hand.   Use these two transitional phrases as a pair. For less wordiness, substitute *yet*, *but*, or *however*.

> Poor: *On one hand, she hoped for a favorable report. On the other hand, she knew her prognosis was guarded.*
> Improved: *She hoped for a favorable report but knew her prognosis was guarded.*

one.   Avoid using the pronoun *one* as the subject of a sentence.

> Poor: *When debating an issue, one should be sure of the facts.*
> Improved: *When debating an issue, be sure of the facts.*

one another.   Use interchangeably with *each other*.

ongoing.   One word. Never hyphenate.

only.   Place *only* **before** the word it modifies.

> *Mary only cared about passing the test.* (Mary cared, but others didn't.)
> *Mary cared only about passing the test.* (Mary didn't care about anything but passing the test.)

operationalize.   Regarded as bureaucratic or corporate jargon. To be avoided. See *ize*.

oral, verbal.   Not interchangeable. *Oral* refers to spoken words; *verbal* refers to the spoken, written, or printed word.

The psychologist gave an oral promise.
His verbal skills will take him far in life.

orient, orientate.   Synonymous verbs meaning "to make familiar" or "to locate." Avoid orientate, a pretentious term, except to mean "to face or turn to the east."

over.   Use to indicate motion or a "position higher than or above another." Not interchangeable with more than.

Poor: *Cynthia Wu worked at her post for over ten years.*

Improved: *Cynthia Wu worked at her post for more than ten years.*

P

pagination.   When preparing a manuscript, begin Arabic numbering on page 2 in the upper right corner, flush with the upper margin. Do not number page 1 unless the publication requests it.

parallelism.   Refers to sentences or phrases in which the elements have the same format or relationships expressed in the same grammatical format.

He relaxes by communing on a mountaintop, snorkling in the Bahamas, and singing in the shower.

Avoid faulty parallelism. Don't use the same grammatical form when the locutions (words or groups of related words) are not logical and parallel.

Poor: *The patient was asked to call the physician's secretary and an appointment would be given.*

Improved: *The patient was asked to call the physician's secretary to make an appointment.*

parameter. Use for mathematical expressions only. Experts dispute the use of parameter in nonmathematical expressions, such as *parameters of practice.* Use *boundary* instead.

parentheses and brackets. Use parentheses normally to surround numbers or letters listing items in a series: *(1) the symptoms, (2) the diagnosis.*

In the first reference to members of Congress, always indicate the political and geographic designation, in parentheses, immediately after the name.

Sen. John Fairweather (D-CT) attended the reception.

Parentheses are also used to enclose loosely related explanations.

Brackets have little use in professional writing. Editorial remarks inserted as explanations within a quote, or a bridging phrase substituted for an omitted portion of a quote should appear in brackets. They are used primarily for stage directions and for enclosing sic within to indicate misspellings in quotes.

Her memo concluded with "Yours Truley [sic],

Sally Chase."

Colette [pacing]: How long must we wait?

participles. See verbals.

payer, payor. Payer, meaning "a payer of bills," is recognized as the proper form. Some medical and nursing journals, however, suggest payor for their style, as in third-party payor.

people, persons. People refers to a group and implies anonymity, except when certain individuals are emphasized. "Persons" refers to unnamed individuals within a group.

Thousands of people attended the banquet.

Luther Kean, Rozella Ford, and Dee Ferguson were among the people invited to the retreat.

Of the 50 people she invited, only 20 persons attended.

per.   A preposition. Two common meanings are "to, for, for every" and "according to."

> *The cardiologist recommended that Fred swim no more than one hour per day.*
>
> *Per instructions of the vice president, the associate directors revised their departmental budgets.*

percent.   Percent takes either a singular or plural verb, depending on its meaning. Per cent is obsolete.

> *The program director said 20 percent was too low a figure.* (singular verb)
>
> *The medical society's statistics show that 40 percent of physicians in the state support the measure.* (plural verb)

percentage.   Use percentage, rather than percent, to indicate a portion or amount.

> *A large percentage of the membership voted to move ahead with the hospital's new total quality management program.*
>
> *A high percentage of the patients on 4C were diagnosed with AIDS.*

Use the word percent, rather than the symbol, in formal writing except in charts, graphs, or tables.

> Poor: *The margin of error is 15%.*
>
> Improved: *The margin of error is 15 percent.*

perk, perquisite.   A perquisite is a benefit. Use perk only in informal writing.

> *One of the perquisites for remaining five years was a substantial Christmas bonus.*
>
> *One of the medical center's perks was free parking.*

phenomenon, phenomena.   Phenomenon is singular, phenomena is plural.

> *Dr. Morton's introduction of ether at Massachusetts General Hospital was considered not only an innovation but an amazing phenomenon.*
>
> *The study of phenomena is an important concept in qualitative research.*

plurals.   Plurals are terms composed of more than one member, set, or kind. Plurals are formed in several ways.

    a. *combined words.* Usually add the s to the first word as in *sisters-in-law, Attorneys General,* or *rights-of-way.* In military titles, however, the s is usually added to the second word as in *lieutenant colonels* or *major generals.*

> *Several editors in chief spoke at the journalism seminar.*

    b. *proper names.* As in simple plurals, merely add an s or es. Names that end in y do not change to ie as in common nouns. Add an s as in *Kennedys.* Exceptions include the mountain chains called the *Rockies* and *Alleghenies.* If a name ends in es or z, add es: *Joneses, Gonzalezes.*

    c. *numerals.* The trend is to omit the apostrophe ('), but be consistent if used.

> *1960s, size 10s, 1920s, 90s, Roaring 20s, in her 30s*

    d. *letters.*   With single letters, use an apostrophe; with multiple letters, no apostrophe.

> *p's   q's   ABCs   IOUs   CEOs   RNs   MDs*

    e. *common nouns.* Add s or es to form plurals, as in *nurses, lenses, glasses.* Add es to words ending in o preceded by a consonant, as in *potatoes* and *heroes,* but not *pianos* or *mottos.*

plus.   A conjunction meaning "increased by the addition of"; a noun meaning "a positive quality"; and an adjective meaning "positive."

> *My salary plus benefits is acceptable.* (conjunction)
> *The administrator's willingness to negotiate is a plus for the institution.* (noun)
> *Faith's ability to communicate well is a plus factor.* (adjective)

possessives.   See apostrophe.

practical, practicable.   Use practical to mean "relating to practice in action," practicable to mean "capable of being done."

> *Theory followed by practical experience is highly desirable.*
> *The model she proposed was too complex to be practicable.*

practicum, practicums.   The preferred plural is practicums, rather than practica.

precipitate, precipitous.   As a verb, precipitate means "to bring about abruptly." As an adjective, it means "moving heedlessly." Precipitous, an adjective, means "steep," like a precipice, but it can be used to mean "hasty, rash, or sudden." It can be synonymous with the adjective precipitate.

> *The patient's noncompliance precipitated an acute attack.*
> *It was a precipitate move to dismiss the staff.*
> *His precipitous decision to close the unit would have serious consequences.*

preventive, preventative.   Interchangeable but preventive is preferred.

primary health care.   Care an individual receives at the first point of contact with the health care system, which may occur in the community, the home, or a health care facility. Emphasis is on a long-term relationship among patient, family, and practitioner.

primary nursing. Care provided in a health care facility in which the nurse is responsible as well as accountable for the overall plan of care of an assigned patient from admission, throughout hospitalization over a 24-hour period, to discharge.

principal, principle. As a noun, principal means "a person of rank" or "a sum of money"; as an adjective, it means "first in rank or importance." Principle, a noun only, is "a basic truth or rule of conduct."

> *The principal concept of her proposal lacked credibility.*
> *The principal closed the school because of inclement weather.*
> *Never compromise your principles.*

prioritize. Not recommended for professional writing, although its use has increased in spoken and written communication. Considered corporate and bureaucratic jargon.

privatize. Same as the preceding entry.

proved, proven. Use proven as an adjective, as in *proven facts.* Use proved only as past participle of the verb to prove.

> *The patient proved (had proven) the physician's culpability.*

Q

quality. Noun. Do not use as an adjective except in compound words such as *quality assurance, quality control,* and *quality point.*

> Poor: *The nurse provided high-quality care.*
> Improved: *The nurse provided care of high quality.*

quasi. An adjective "having some resemblance usually by possession of certain attributes."

The National League for Nursing is a quasi-professional nursing organization.

quotation marks. Place periods and commas within quotation marks. Place colons and semicolons outside quotation marks.

Danielle's most telling comment was that "the person who thinks clearly, writes clearly."

She defined "burnout": a phenomenon created by overextended individuals.

Question marks and exclamation points may come before or after quotation marks, depending on the meaning.

Have you ever read "The Universal Declaration of Human Rights"?

As the speaker left the podium, he called out, "Hail and farewell!"

When a paragraph of quoted material is followed by another paragraph that continues the quotation, do not end the first paragraph with an end quote ("). Begin the second paragraph with an open quote and use the end quote only at the end of the quoted material.

Quoted material exceeding three lines in a paragraph should be indented in block form **without** quotation marks.

quote, quotation. Use quotation to mean "a passage that is quoted from a speech or work." Quote is acceptable in speech, not in formal writing. As a verb, quote means "to repeat a passage from another work."

Poor: *The following quote illustrates my point.*

Improved: *The following quotation illustrates my point.*

R

raised, reared.   Only humans are reared; any living thing can be raised.

rape.   Term preferred to criminal attack, criminal assault, sexual assault, and other general terms.

record.   When used as a noun, avoid the redundant new record.

Poor: *She set a new record for promptness.*

Improved: *She set a record for promptness.*

Acceptable: *His new record surpassed the old.*

referencing.   By documenting a written work, you credit the source. You add to the credibility of the discussion in progress because, by their very nature, citations clue in your readers to the effectiveness of the supporting evidence. You document by developing your list of sources and by providing references—usually parenthetical—in the text that are consistent with the list.

If you intend to publish, your best bet is to obtain the style requirements of the journals or publishing companies to which you may wish to submit your work. Check the journals in the health care area, since many carry author guidelines on a regular basis and are quite clear as to reference specifications. You also may write directly to specific publications for the information.

Although a number of editors follow the general pattern of academia, which tends to favor the *Publication Manual of the American Psychological Association* (3d edition, 1988 printing), others use different sources or develop their own eclectic approach to referencing. Writers of monographs and similar works, in which no particular format is suggested, should choose the style most comfortable for them. Gehle and Rollo (1987) offer some excellent tips on how to cite correctly when using different types of references.

Whatever style you use in professional writing, always follow three rules in documenting:

1. Make it clear.
2. Make it complete.
3. Make it accurate.

regarding.   Synonymous for <u>about</u>, <u>concerning</u>, or <u>on</u>.

regardless, irregardless.   Use <u>regardless</u> to mean "in spite of." Irre-gardless is not a word.

regime, regimen.   Not interchangeable. Use <u>regime</u> to mean "a system of management" and <u>regimen</u> for "a system of therapy."

> *Case management was the accepted regime at her hospital.*
> *The physician put the patient on a low-salt, low-cholesterol regimen.*

regretful, regrettable.   Not interchangeable. Use regretful to mean "full of regret, sorry" and regrettable to mean "deserving regret."

> *Dr. Casey was regretful about the misunderstanding with his staff.*
> *The entire incident was regrettable because two of his assistants misinterpreted the order.*

relative (to).   Means "pertinent to" or "relevant to." Not synonymous with "regarding."

> Poor: *Ms. Mahoney spoke relative to the graduate program.*
> Improved: *Ms. Mahoney's remarks were relative to the goals of the graduate program.*

research, study.   As a noun, use <u>research</u> to mean "a scholarly inquiry or investigation." As a verb, it means "to search or investigate exhaustively." Do not use as an adjective except as part of a compound term: <u>research grant</u>, <u>research assistant</u>. As a noun, <u>study</u> means "pursuit of knowledge." Not all studies are research, but all research involves a study. The term "research study" is redundant. Avoid.

> Poor: *She conducted her research study on patients housed in the surgical intensive care unit.*
>
> Improved: *She conducted her research (or study) on patients housed in the surgical intensive care unit.*

S

Saint.   Abbreviate as St. before the name of a saint and in names of cities and other places. Exceptions exist, particularly with names of hospitals. Check the source.

semicolon.   Overused punctuation mark. Use to create a more significant break in lieu of a comma, such as in compound sentences and between independent clauses not joined by a connecting word.

> *The committee determined several issues to be explored at the nursing retreat: advancing the education base; standardizing certification; implementing the agenda for health care reform; and improving the profession's visibility.*
>
> *Giving injections, particularly to children, was one of Ms. Shott's least favorite tasks; nevertheless it became a challenge.*

serve, service.   Both mean "to provide a service" but they are not interchangeable. People are served; inanimate objects are serviced.

> *The aide served the patient his dinner.*
>
> *The electrician serviced the equipment in the patient's room.*

sexist language.   Whenever possible, use the plural form to avoid the generic use of masculine or feminine pronouns. If inappropriate, employ the gender representing the majority of the group or category described. Avoid use of he/she or his/her unless a publication for which you are writing requests this usage.

Poor: *A health professional cannot use knowledge that he doesn't have.*

Improved: *Health professionals cannot use knowledge that they don't have.*

shall, will.   To express simple futurity, use shall in the first person and will in the second and third persons.

We (I) shall go to the hemodynamics workshop.
You (he) will go to the hemodynamics workshop.

To express determination, promise, or command, use will in the first person, and shall in the second and third persons.

We will.
You shall.

should, would.   Use should in all persons in place of the present subjunctive. Use would in all persons to express determination or habitual action.

Even if I (you, she) should fail the test, the instructor would be fair.
She cautioned me, but I would have my way.
He would consult with the therapist each week to ascertain his progress.

simile.   See figurative language.

since, because.   Synonymous only when used as conjunctions.

He typed the letter on his old manual Underwood since (because) his computer printer broke down.
The staff has been delighted since the administration decided to decentralize the nursing service to the unit level.

sometime, sometimes.   Both adverbs. Sometime means "at an indefinite time"; sometimes means "upon occasion."

> *Oliver planned to obtain his master's degree sometime in the future.*
> *Sometimes Oliver was sorry that he didn't return to school sooner.*

split infinitives.   See verbals.

state.   Lowercase state when it refers to a specific jurisdiction standing alone. Capitalize when it refers to a state's government.

> *Hank was concerned about environmental problems in his state.*
> *The State of Florida applied for federal assistance to cover hurricane damage.*

stationary, stationery.   Use stationary to mean "fixed, motionless," stationery to mean "writing material."

staunch, stanch.   Use staunch, an adjective, to mean "steadfast and true." Use stanch, a verb, to mean "to stop a flow of liquid, such as blood."

stratum, strata.   Strata, or sometimes stratums, is preferred to stratas as the plural.

supine, prone.   Don't confuse meanings on these adjectives. Supine means "face up," prone means "face down."

syllabus, syllabuses.   Use syllabuses, rather than syllabi as the plural.

T

that, which.   Relative pronouns. When used in restrictive clauses (essential for the meaning of the sentence), that is preferable. Use *which* with nonrestrictive clauses. Set off nonrestrictive (non-essential) clauses with commas.

> *When she attended the cardiac symposium that took place in her hometown, the event was more exciting for her.*
>
> *The maximum dosage, which must not exceed 150 mg bid, still creates some serious side effects.*

this, those, these, that.   Demonstrative pronouns. Use sparingly.

> Poor: *This is the way Dr. Stych wants the technique performed.*
> Improved: *This technique is Dr. Stych's preference.*

through, thru.   A variation of through, the word thru should not be used in formal writing.

time.   Use numerals in stating a time: 9:20 A.M. Avoid using 9 o'clock, as well as redundant terms such as *9:20 A.M. this morning* or *at 3:30 P.M. yesterday afternoon.* A.M. and P.M. can be capitals or lower case, with or without periods, but be consistent.

to, too.   To is a preposition showing direction. The adverb too means "also."

> *Doris went promptly to the luncheon.*
>
> *We have delayed a decision too long to accomplish our goals.*

toward, to.   Use toward to mean "in the direction of," to "in a direction toward."

> *The nurse managers walked **toward** the conference room on their way **to** rounds.*

TV.   Use television rather than the abbreviation in professional writing.

U

under way.   Two words.

Planning for the new facility is under way.

unique.   "The only one of its kind." Not synonymous with unusual.

The practitioner-teacher role, with its combined components of education and practice, is a unique concept in American nursing.

universal precautions.   Lowercase.

up to date.   Hyphenate only as an adjective.

He used up-to-date references for his talk.
She kept her financial records up to date.

usage, use.   Usage refers to "habitual or preferred practices." Use shows "employment or usefulness."

Good writers strive to master proper language usage.
Sheila's use of a styleguide increased her chances to publish.

United States.   Abbreviate only as an adjective in names of government agencies, such as U.S. Department of Commerce, in designations of highways, and in quoted material. United States is singular. The possessive is *United States'*.

V

verb agreement.   A verb always agrees with its subject, not with modifiers or introductory phrases.

Here come Professor Block and the teaching assistant.
Here comes Ms. Smiley, the clinical specialist.

A verb agrees with its subject, not the expletive there.

There are many reasons for Chuck Swift's promotion.

Singular subjects joined by or or nor take singular verbs.

The social worker could not determine whether the child or the mother was responsible.
Neither Lucille nor her brother was hospitalized.

When a singular and plural subject are joined by or or nor, the verb agrees with the nearest word.

The clinical coordinator does not know whether the staff nurses or the aide is responsible for the error.

The indefinite pronouns each and every and compound subjects modified by each and every take singular verbs.

Each of the therapists is bringing his own recommendation.
Each bedside unit has its own computer.
Every room and suite is equipped with the latest technology.

Collective nouns can take singular or plural verbs, depending on whether they are considered a singular unit or as individuals in a group.

The committee is meeting tomorrow. (collective)
The committee are arriving for the meeting. (individuals)
The staff is meeting now. (singular unit)
The staff are being evaluated on Friday. (individuals)

The antecedent of the relative pronoun (who, which, or that) determines the number and person of the verb of which the pronoun is the subject.

It is I who am accountable.

It is you who deserve the praise.

She is one of those progressive administrators who advocate participatory management. (Verb is plural to agree with administrators)

no one, anyone, everyone, and someone; nobody, anybody, everybody, and somebody—all require singular verbs.

No one was prepared to assign responsibility because everyone was culpable.

verb usage:

a. *choosing the exact verb.* Good writing requires choosing exact words to convey immediately and accurately a complex idea. Weak and common verbs like look, walk, and go can often be replaced by concrete verbs that show the action more vividly and exactly. Consider these examples:

Poor: *The patient walked down the hall in an unsteady way.*

Improved: *The patient tottered (or staggered—or whatever he did) down the hall.*

Poor: *He looked at the psychologist in an angry way.*

Improved: *He glowered (or glared) at the psychologist.*

Poor: *She made funny faces as the doctor described her options.*

Improved: *She grimaced as the doctor described her options.*

b. *accentuate the positive.* Active verbs will give vitality to your writing. Whenever possible, avoid passive voice.

Poor: *It is expected that you will follow the protocol.*

Improved: *We expect you to follow the protocol.*

Poor: *The student was reassured by her instructor's confident manner.*

Improved: *The instructor's confident manner reassured the student.*

Poor: *When Elizabeth was queen . . . .*
Improved: *When Elizabeth reigned . . . .*

c. *weed out weak-linking verbs.* Verbs such as is, have, and other forms of "to be" tend to generate lazy prose and produce tedious writing. Try to overcome this pitfall.

Poor: *The treatment will be for six weeks and should then be effective.*
Improved: *The six-week treatment should prove effective.*

Poor: *Frances can be on the dean's list if her grades are good.*
Improved: *Frances can make the dean's list if she maintains good grades.*

d. *keep your verbs as verbs.* Maintaining the integrity of your verbs is an important principle to follow in all types of writing. Avoid the practice of converting verbs into nouns with endings such as -tion, -tize, -ance, -ability, and -able.

Poor: *Hospital officials agreed on the implementation of the new orientation program.*
Improved: *Hospital officials agreed to implement the new orientation program.*

Poor: *Don gave an unconvincing explanation for his tardiness.*
Improved: *Don explained unconvincingly his tardiness.*

Some other common examples are as follows:

Verb	Abstract Noun
advance	advancement of
determine	determination
excite	excitability
govern	governance
use	utilization

e. *excessive predication.* Avoid using more verbs than necessary.

Poor: *The visitor entered the patient's room, which was filled with flowers.*

Improved: *The visitor entered the patient's flower-filled room.*

verbals. A verbal is a verb used as a noun, adjective, or adverb. A verbal may be a gerund, participle, or infinitive.

a. *gerund.* A verbal created by adding -ing to a verb; used as a noun, while conveying the meaning of a verb.

Editing (from to edit) *becomes easier when using a styleguide.*

b. *participle.* A verbal formed by adding -ing is a present participle. Past participles end in -d, -ed, -n, -en, or t (unless the verb changes form altogether, such as sung). Participles are used as adjectives.

Smiling, Dorothy accepted her colleague's thanks.
Embarrassed by her faux pas, she tried to recover her composure.

Avoid adding -ing to popular words to produce senseless verbals.

Poor: *dialoguing with peers*
Improved: *conversing (or talking) with peers*

Poor: *servicing clients*
Improved: *helping clients*

c. *infinitive.* A verbal with to in front of the verb.

To err is human. (subject)
Ms. Huffnagle loves to work on her computer. (direct object)

This conference is the one to attend. (adjective)

Nelson's disposition was difficult to tolerate. (adverb modifying difficult)

versus.   Do not abbreviate as vs in professional writing. Use the abbreviation v when referring to court cases, as in *Smith v Davenport.*

> *It was nurses versus medical residents in the doubles tournament.*

very, rather.   Avoid using these adverbs to strengthen an adjective.

> Poor: *very big*
> Improved: *massive, huge*

> Poor: *rather touchy*
> Improved: *sensitive, ticklish*

vice.   As a prefix, the use of the hyphen is optional. The trend is to drop the hyphen.

> *vice-president, vice president*

victim.   Avoid using victim to refer to a patient with a disease or disability. See also Section V, B.

> Poor: *AIDS victim*
> Improved: *Person with AIDS*

viz.   See Latin derivatives.

W

whether.   Implies an alternative. Rarely needs to be followed by or not.

who, whom, whose, which. Relative pronouns. Use who to mean "he, she, or they."

> *Judith Springsley, who joined the firm in January, was a refreshing addition to the staff.*

Use whom to mean "him, her, or them."

> *Marion Rodriquez, whom the committee recommended, began the task immediately.*

Use whose (or of whom or of which) to express the possessive.

> *The committee, whose last recommendation was rejected by the board, supported the appointment of Ms. Rodriquez.*

Use which to describe an impersonal object or thing.

> *He was impressed by the group, which identified goals for the future.*

who, whose, which, what. As interrogative pronouns, they are used to introduce a direct or indirect question.

> *Who wants to go on grand rounds?* (direct question)
> *The clinical specialist wondered who had ordered the consultation.* (indirect)

X

x ray, x-ray. Hyphenate as an adjective or transitive verb, not as a noun.

> *The x ray should be taken as soon as possible.* (noun)
> *The x-ray therapy was successful.* (adjective)
> *The technician x-rayed him at home.* (verb)

Y

years.   Use numerals to express years. Avoid beginning a sentence with a numeral. Rather than write out the numeral, rework the sentence.

Poor: *1984 was a good year.*
Improved: *A good year was 1984.*

Set off the year with a comma when presenting a full date.

We opened the new hospital on January 5, 1993.

No comma is necessary if no specific date is given.

We opened the new hospital in January 1993.

Combine successive years with a hyphen. Use 1993–94 rather than 1993–1994.

Her annual report covered the period 1991–92.

Use an apostrophe to form the shorter form of a year as in more informal contexts.

The class of '93 won top honors.

Z

zero. Write out *zero* in sentences where no other numeral is used.

The committee discussed zero-based budgeting.

Use a unit of measurement when zero is written as a numeral.

The incidence of the disease rose from 0 percent to six percent in three months.

ZIP code.   Acronym for Z(one) I(mprovement) P(rogram). When writing a mailing address, do not insert a comma between the state abbreviation (always in capital letters) and the ZIP code.

Springfield, MA 95302

II

Interpret Those Abbreviations/Acronyms

Although people tend to confuse abbreviations and acronyms, the terms are not synonymous. An abbreviation is a shortened form of a written word or phrase used in place of the whole. Examples include APHA (American Public Health Association), and CPR (cardiopulmonary resuscitation).

An acronym is a word formed from the initial or key letter or letters of each of a series of words. RUGS (research utilization groups) and CHAP (Community Health Accreditation Program) are classified as acronyms. Acronyms may include adjoining letters to make them pronounceable.

The listing below combines abbreviations and acronyms. Part A includes the more common terms used by health professionals. Part B represents a compendium of the more familiar organizations and agencies.

For a complete directory of nursing organizations as well as government health-related bodies, check the annual April issue of the *American Journal of Nursing*. Abbreviations and acronyms, however, do not appear in the majority of the *AJN* entries.

A. Abbreviations/Acronyms in the Nursing and Health Field

ABE	acute bacterial endocarditis
ABS	acute brain syndrome
ACLS	advanced cardiac life support
ACS	ambulatory care services
ACT	added compensatory time
ACVD	acute cardiovascular disease
A & D	admission and discharge
AD	admitting diagnosis
AD	after discharge
ADC	average daily census
ADHC	adult day health care
ADL	activities of daily living
AD/LIB	freely
ADN	associate degree in nursing
ADP	automatic data processing
ADR	actual death rate
ADR	adverse drug reaction
ADS	alternative delivery system
ADT	admission/discharge/transfer
AEC	at earliest convenience
AIDS	acquired immune deficiency syndrome
AL	arterial line
ALC	allowable limits of care
ALC	alternate levels of care
ALOH	average length of hospitalization
ALOS	average length of stay
ALS	advanced life support
AMA	against medical advice

AMI	*acute myocardial infarction*
AND	*administratively necessary days*
ANDA	*abbreviated new drug application*
ANOV	*analysis of variance*
AOB	*adjusted occupied bed*
A & P	*assessment and plans*
APG	*ambulatory patient groups*
A/R	*apical/radial*
ASAP	*as soon as possible*
ASF	*ambulatory surgical facility*
ATLS	*advanced trauma life support*
AWD	*absent without discharge*
BB	*blood bank*
BC	*board certified*
BID	*twice daily*
BLC	*basic life support*
BM	*bone marrow*
BM	*bowel movement*
BMR	*basal metabolic rate*
BMT	*bone marrow transplant*
BP	*bed pan*
BP	*blood pressure*
BR	*bedrest*
BRN	*board of registered nursing* (state specific)
BRN	*baccalaureate program for registered nurse*
BRP	*bathroom privileges*
BSN	*bachelor of science in nursing*
BSN	*bowel sounds normal*
BT	*bedtime*
BU	*burn unit*
C	*certified*

CA	*carcinoma (or cancer)*
CABG	*coronary artery bypass graft*
CAI	*computer assisted instruction*
CAPD	*continuous ambulatory peritoneal dialysis*
CAR	*computer assisted retrieval*
CAT	*computerized adaptive testing*
CBC	*complete blood count*
CBF	*cerebral blood flow*
CBVI	*computer-based video instruction*
CC	*chief complaint*
CC	*conventional care*
CC	*critical care*
CCP	*comprehensive care plan*
CCU	*coronary care unit*
CCU	*critical care unit*
CD	*cardiovascular disease*
CDU	*chemical dependency unit*
CE	*continuing education*
CEA	*cost-effective analysis*
CEO	*chief executive officer*
CEU	*continuing education unit*
CFO	*chief financial officer*
CHC	*community health center*
CHCP	*coordinated home care program*
CHI	*consumer health information*
CHIP	*comprehensive health insurance plan*
CHN	*community health network*
CIO	*chief information officer*
CIS	*computer information service*
CM	*case management*
CM	*case mix*

CMI	*case mix index*
CMP	*comprehensive medical plan*
CNAA	*certified nursing administrator, advanced*
CNE	*chief nurse executive*
CNM	*certified nurse-midwife*
CNP	*community nurse practitioner*
CNS	*clinical nurse specialist*
C/O	*complaint of*
COO	*chief operating officer*
COI	*cost of illness*
CON	*certificate of need*
COPD	*chronic obstructive pulmonary disease*
CPM	*continuous passive motion*
CPO	*continuous pulse oximetry*
CPR	*cardiopulmonary resuscitation*
CPU	*central processing unit*
CQI	*continuous quality improvement*
CRF	*case report form*
CRNA	*certified registered nurse anesthetist*
CRT	*cardiac resuscitation team*
CSDS	*corporate strategic planning system*
CSR	*central supply room*
CSW	*clinical social worker*
CT	*computerized axial tomography*
CVL	*central venous line*
CVP	*central venous pressure*
D/A	*date of admission*
D/C	*discontinue*
DD	*dual degree*
DDS	*doctor of dental surgery*
DHS	*duration of hospital stay*

DNA	*district nurses association*
DNI	*do not intubate*
DNR	*do not resuscitate*
DNS	*doctor of nursing science*
DNSc	*doctor of nursing science*
DOA	*date of admission*
DOA	*dead on arrival*
DON	*director of nursing*
DOQ	*desired order quantity*
DP	*data processing*
DR	*delivery room*
DRG	*diagnosis related group*
DRS	*data retrieval system*
DSN	*doctor of science in nursing*
E & A	*evaluate and advise*
ECF	*extended care facility*
ECG, EKG	*electrocardiography*
ECT	*electroconvulsive therapy*
ECU	*extended care unit*
ED	*emergency department*
EdD	*doctor of education*
EDP	*electronic data processing*
EDR	*expected death rate*
EEG	*electroencephalography*
EEO	*equal employment opportunity*
EMT	*emergency medical team*
EOC	*episode of care*
ER	*emergency room*
ESRD	*end stage renal disease*
FAAN	*fellow of the American Academy of Nursing*
FFS	*fee for service*

FHC	*family health center*
FHIP	*family health insurance plan*
FI	*fiscal intermediary*
FNP	*family nurse practitioner*
FTE	*full time equivalent*
FUO	*fever of unknown origin*
FY	*fiscal year*
GN	*graduate nurse*
GNP	*gerontologic (geriatric) nurse practitioner*
GNTR	*graduate nurse transition program*
GR	*grand rounds*
GRE	*graduate record examination*
HB	*hospital-based*
HBO	*health benefits organization*
HBP	*hospital-based physician*
HBV	*hepatitis B virus*
HC	*health care*
HCD	*health care delivery*
HH	*home hyperalimentation*
HHA	*home health agency*
HHA	*home health aide*
HHC	*home health care*
HIP	*health insurance plan*
HIS	*home information system*
HIV	*human immunodeficiency virus*
HMO	*health maintenance organization*
HN	*head nurse*
HO	*house officer*
HOPA	*hospital-based organ procurement agency*
HP	*health professional*
HP	*house physician*

HPN	*home parenteral nutrition*
HPPD	*hours per patient day*
HPR	*hospital peer review*
HR	*hospital record*
HR	*human resources*
HSC	*health science center*
HSI	*health status index*
IC	*intensive care*
ICF	*intermediate care facility*
ICP	*intercranial pressure*
ICU	*intensive care unit*
IDS	*interactive data system*
I/O	*intake/output*
IV	*intravenous*
IVP	*intravenous pyelogram*
KCF	*key clinical finding*
MAP	*mean arterial pressure*
MASH	*mobile army surgical hospital*
MBA	*master of business administration*
MC	*managed care*
MCH	*maternal and child health*
MCN	*maternal child nursing*
MD	*doctor of medicine*
MDC	*major diagnostic category*
MDS	*minimum data set*
MHA	*master of health administration*
MI	*myocardial infarction*
MIC	*maternal and infant care*
MICU	*medical intensive care unit*
MIS	*management information system*
MIS	*medical information system*

MPH	*master of public health*
MPP	*Medicare-participating physician*
MPS	*multiphasic screening*
MR	*management review*
MR	*mental retardation*
MRA	*multiple regression analysis*
MRI	*magnetic resonance imaging*
MSDS	*material safety data sheet*
MSN	*master of science in nursing*
MSW	*master of social work*
NA	*not admitted*
NA	*notice of admission*
NA	*nursing assistant (or aide)*
NAC	*nursing audit committee*
NCLEX	*National Council Licensure Examination*
NFP	*not for profit*
NICU	*neonatal intensive care unit*
NICU	*neurosurgical intensive care unit*
NIS	*nursing information system*
NG	*nasogastric*
NM	*nurse manager*
NMIS	*nursing management information system*
NNP	*neonatal nurse practitioner*
NP	*nurse practitioner*
NPO	*nothing by mouth*
NRC	*nursing resource cluster*
NSA	*nursing service administrator*
NSAIDS	*nonsteroidal anti-inflammatory drugs*
NTA	*nurse training act*
NTBR	*not to be resuscitated*
OBS	*organic brain syndrome*

OCU	*outpatient care unit*
OD	*organizational development*
OJT	*on-the-job training*
OOB	*out of bed*
OPA	*organ procurement agency*
OPD	*outpatient department*
ORS	*outpatient surgery*
OR	*operating room*
OR	*organ recovery*
OTC	*over the counter*
OTR	*registered occupational therapist*
PA	*physician's assistant*
PAC	*political action committee*
PAP	*patient assessment program*
PAR	*postanesthesia room*
PARU	*postanesthesia recovery unit*
PCO$_2$	*partial pressure carbon dioxide*
PCS	*patient care clinicians*
PD	*patient day*
PDR	*Physician's Desk Reference*
PEC	*patient education coordinator*
PET	*positron emission tomography*
PGP	*prepaid group practice*
PHC	*primary health care*
PhD	*doctor of philosophy*
PHO	*physician hospital organization*
PNP	*pediatric nurse practitioner*
PO$_2$	*partial pressure oxygen*
PPO	*preferred provided organization*
PPS	*prospective payment system*
PR	*peer review*

PRO	peer review organization
PRS	prospective reimbursement system
PSDA	patient self-determination act
PT	physical therapist
PTA	prior to admission
PTCA	percutaneous transluminal coronary angioplasty
QA & I	quality assurance and improvement
QAP	quality assurance program
QC	quality circle
QD	every day
QHS	every hour of sleep
QID	four times a day
QPC	quality of patient care
QPM	every night
QWL	quality of work life
RC	referred care
R & D	research and development
RD	registered dietitian
RFI	request for information
RFP	request for proposal
RIMS	relative intensity measures
RM	risk management
RN	registered nurse
RNC	registered nurse certified
RNLP	registered nurse, license pending
R & R	rest and recuperation/relaxation
RR	recovery room
RT	respiratory therapist
RUGS	research utilization groups
RVS	relative value scales
RVU	relative value unit

SBE	*subacute bacterial endocarditis*
SBN	*state board of nursing*
SCU	*special care unit*
SG	*Surgeon General*
SI	*seriously ill*
SICU	*surgical intensive care unit*
SN	*staff nurse*
SNA	*state nurses association*
SNF	*skilled nursing facility*
SO	*significant other*
SOC	*standard of care*
SOI	*severity of illness*
SOP	*standard operating procedure*
SP	*standard performance*
SPA	*state planning agency*
SVCS	*superior vena cava syndrome*
SW	*social worker*
TC	*transplant center*
TID	*three times daily*
TLC	*tender loving care*
TPN	*total parenteral nutrition*
TQM	*total quality management*
TR	*turnover rate*
TRO	*temporary restraining order*
TT	*turnover time*
U & A	*up and about*
UCRS	*utilization control reporting system*
UCS	*usual and customary service*
UD	*unit dose*
UOS	*units of service*
UR	*utilization review*

URI	upper respiratory infection
VNA	visiting nurse association
VNS	visiting nurse service
VP	vice president
VS	vital signs
WCH	women and children's health
WL	workload
WNL	within normal limits
YACP	young adult chronic patient
YTD	yes-to-date
ZBB	zero-based budgeting
ZPG	zero population growth

B. Selected Abbreviations/Acronyms of Nursing and Health-Related Organizations and Agencies

AA	Alcoholics Anonymous
AAA	American Aging Association
AAAS	American Association for the Advancement of Science
AACN	American Association of Colleges of Nursing
AACN	American Association of Critical Care Nurses
AAJCC	American Association of Junior and Community Colleges
AAMC	American Association of Medical Colleges
AAN	American Academy of Nursing
AANP	American Academy of Nurse Practitioners
AAP	American Association of Pediatrics
AARP	American Association of Retired Persons
ABMS	American Board of Medical Specialties

ABNS	*American Board of Nursing Specialties*
ACGME	*Accreditation Council for Graduate Medical Education*
ACHA	*American College Health Association*
ACHE	*American College of Health Care Executives*
ACLU	*American Civil Liberties Union*
ACNHA	*American College of Nursing Home Administrators*
ACNM	*American College of Nurse-Midwives*
ACP	*American College of Physicians*
ACS	*American Cancer Society*
ACSW	*Academy of Certified Social Workers*
ADA	*American Dental Association*
ADAMA	*Alcohol, Drug Abuse, and Mental Health Administration*
AF	*Arthritis Foundation*
AFNC	*Air Force Nurse Corps*
AHA	*American Heart Association*
AHA	*American Hospital Association*
AHCA	*American Health Care Association*
AHCPR	*Agency for Health Care Policy and Research*
AHFS	*American Hospital Formulary Service*
AHPA	*American Health Planning Association*
AHSR	*Association for Health Services Research*
AIHCA	*American Indian Health Care Association*
AJN(CO)	*American Journal of Nursing Company*
AMA	*American Medical Association*
ANA	*American Nurses Association*
ANC	*Army Nurse Corps*
ANF	*American Nurses Foundation*
AOA	*Administration on Aging*

AONE	Association of Nurse Executives
AORN	Association of Operating Room Nurses
AOTA	American Occupational Therapy Association
APA	American Pharmaceutical Association
APA	American Psychiatric Association
APA	American Psychological Association
APHA	American Public Health Association
ARC	American Red Cross
ASA	American Society on Aging
ASAHP	American Society of Allied Health Professionals
ASHA	American School Health Association
ASHP	American Society for Hospital Pharmacists
ASHRM	American Society for Hospital Risk Management
ASIM	American Society of Internal Medicine
BLS	Bureau of Labor Statistics
CDC	Centers for Disease Control and Prevention
CDF	Children's Defense Fund
CHA	Catholic Health Association of the United States
CHAMPUS	Civilian Health and Medical Program of the Uniformed Services
CHAP	Community Health Accreditation Program
COGFNS	Commission on Graduates of Foreign Nursing Schools
COPA	Commission on Post Secondary Accreditation
COTH	Council of Teaching Hospitals
CPEHS	Consumer Protection and Environmental Health Service
DEA	Drug Enforcement Administration

DHHS	Department of Health and Human Services
EEOC	Equal Employment Opportunity Commission
ENRS	Eastern Nursing Research Society
EPA	Environmental Protection Agency
FDA	Food and Drug Administration
FNS	Frontier Nursing Service
FRACHE	Federation of Regional Accrediting Commissions of Higher Education
GSA	Gerontological Society of America
HCA	Hospital Corporation of America
HCFA	Health Care Financing Administration
HFMA	Health Care Financial Management Association
HRSA	Health Resources and Services Administration
ICN	International Council of Nurses
IHI	International Hospital Federation
IHS	Indian Health Service
INANE	International Academy of Nursing Editors
IOM	Institute of Medicine
JCAHO	Joint Commission on the Accreditation of Healthcare Organizations
MAIN	Midwest Alliance in Nursing
MCA	Maternity Center Association
MLA	Medical Library Association
MNRS	Midwest Nursing Research Society
NAACOG	The Organization for Obstetric, Gynecological, and Neonatal Nurses
NAHC	National Association for Home Care
NAHHA	National Association of Home Health Agencies

NANP	National Alliance of Nurse Practitioners
NANR	National Association of Nurse Recruiters
NAP	National Academies of Practice
NAPNAP	National Association of Pediatric Nurse Associates and Practitioners
NAPNES	National Association of Practical Nurse Education and Service
NAPT	National Association of Physical Therapists
NAS	National Academy of Science
NASW	National Association of Social Workers
NCHCA	National Commission for Health Certifying Agencies
NCHCT	National Center for Health Care Technology
NCHPD	National Council of Health Planning and Development
NCHR	National Center for Health Services Research
NCHS	National Center for Health Statistics
NCI	National Cancer Institute
NCOA	National Council of the Aging
NCPI	Nursing Career Reference Inventory
NCPIE	National Council of Patient Information and Education
NCSBN	National Council of State Boards of Nursing
NEA	National Education Association
NEF	Nurses Educational Fund
NEHA	National Environmental Health Association
NEON	Northeast Organization for Nursing
NF	National Foundation
NFLPN	National Federation of Licensed Practical Nurses

NFSNO	National Federation for Specialty Nursing Organizations
NHC	National Health Council
NIA	National Institute on Aging
NIH	National Institutes of Health
NINR	National Institute of Nursing Research
NIOSH	National Institute for Occupational Safety and Health
NLM	National Library of Medicine
NLN	National League for Nursing
NLRB	National Labor Relations Board
NMA	National Medical Association
NMHA	National Mental Health Association
NNC	Navy Nurse Corps
NOLF	Nursing Organizations Liaison Forum
NOW	National Organization for Women
NSF	National Science Foundation
NSNA	National Student Nurses Association
NWHN	National Women's Health Network
ONS	Oncology Nursing Society
OSHA	Occupational Safety and Health Administration
PHA	Premier Hospitals Alliance
PPA	Planned Parenthood Association
PROPAC	Prospective Payment Assessment Commission
SCCN	Southern Collegiate Council on Nursing
SNRS	Southern Nursing Research Society
SRNEF	Society for Research in Nursing Education Forum
SSA	Social Security Administration
STTI	Sigma Theta Tau International

UN	*United Nations*
UNICEF	*United Nations International Children's Emergency Fund*
USPHS	*United States Public Health Service*
VA	*Veterans Administration*
VHA	*Voluntary Hospitals of America*
WHO	*World Health Organization*
WIC	*Women, Infants, and Children's Program*
WIN	*Western Institute of Nursing*
WSNR	*Western Society for Research in Nursing*

III

Simplify Your Language

Long ago Alexander Pope characterized wordiness as follows:

Words are like leaves; and where they most abound
Much fruit of sense beneath is rarely found.

From *An Essay of Criticism*

Scientific language is acceptable as well as necessary, when writing to an audience of peers who will understand such terms like *arteriotomy, palliation,* or *splenic sequestration.* At the same time, use these terms cautiously. Remember that it is better to use *red* in lieu of *erythematous* in most professional writing and it is a "must" for a consumer audience.

A. Watch for Overused Words

The following words are frequently overused by writers. Although they are legitimate and at times may even seem more acceptable, an entire manuscript with too many of them sounds pretentious. Most of the alternative terms listed below are synonymous with the overworked word. Your selection will depend on the use of the word in a sentence.

Keep in mind that these words can be eliminated by merely rephrasing the sentence. Your goal is to make your prose clear and easy to understand for the reader.

Overused Word	Alternative
abbreviate	shorten
accelerate	hasten
accomplish	carry out
accordingly	therefore
accountable	responsible, answerable
actuate	put into action, move
additional	added
aggregate	total
agitate	shake, stir, excite
alleviate	make easier
ameliorate	improve
anticipate	expect
antithesis	opposite
append	add
appropriate (adj.)	proper (adj.)
approximately	about
ascertain	find out
assimilate	absorb, digest
autonomous	independent, self-governing
beneficial	helpful
bilateral	two-sided
bottom line	final result, outcome
burnout	fatigue, exhaustion
circuitous	roundabout
coagulate	thicken
cognizant	aware
commence	begin
commodious	roomy
conception	thought, idea
conjecture	guess
consequently	so
considerable	much

Overused Word	*Alternative*
contiguous	touching, near
criterion	rule, test
deficiency	lack
development	growth
deviate	turn aside
diminution	lessening
empower	enable, authorize
encounter	meet
facilitate	help
hence	so
indeed	in fact
indicate	show
ineffectual	useless
initiate	start, begin
innocuous	harmless
interface	communicate, interact
interrupt	hinder, stop
inundate	flood
isolate	apart
judicious	wise
liberate	free
likewise	and, also
lots, lots of	a great many
lucid	clear
luminous	bright
manifest	clear, plain
manufacture	make
meaningful	important, significant (if not overused)
minimal	smallest
mitigate	make mild, soften
modification	change
moreover	now, next
nebulous	hazy, vague
neutralize	offset
objective	aim, goal
oblique	slanting

Overused Word	*Alternative*
observation	remark
observe	note
obsolete	out-of-date
occupy	take up, fill
operate	work, run
orifice	opening, hole
paradigm	pattern
paramount	top, chief
partially	partly
penetrate	pierce
periphery	outer edge
present (verb)	give
problematical	doubtful
procure	get
purchase	buy
restructure	rebuild, reorganize, revamp
significant	important, striking, telling
super (slang)	wonderful, ideal, first-rate
terminated	died, ended, dismissed
thus	so
utilize	use

B. Watch for Extra Words

Avoid	*Preferred*
a large number	many
a majority of	most
afford the opportunity	permit, allow
ahead of schedule	early
almost never	seldom
are of the opinion	believe
as of now	today
as to	about
at this point in time	now
be kind enough	please

Avoid	*Preferred*
because of the fact that	because
comes in conflict with	conflicts
despite the fact that	although
due in large measure to	due largely to
during the time that	when
except for the fact that	except that
for the purpose of	for
for the reason that	since, because
for this reason	so
give encouragement to	encourage
give rise to	create
had occasion to be	was
in accordance with	according to
in advance of	before
in an impatient manner	impatiently
in favor of	for
in order to	to
in reference to	about
in the event that	if
in the nature of	like
in the near future	soon
in the neighborhood of	about
in the process of (preparing)	preparing
in view of the fact that	since
inasmuch as	since, because
it is often the case that	frequently
it is the intent	we (I) hope
of a confidential nature	confidentially
on account of	because
on the basis of	based on
on the grounds that	since, because
prior to	before
refer back to	refer to
take into consideration	consider
that is to say	in other words
to be sure	of course

Avoid	*Preferred*
until such time as	until, when
with regard to	regarding
with the result that	so that

C. Streamline Your Sentences

Try to write your sentences in crisp and concise language. Think of verbosity as the "curse" of the amateur and remember that a thought in its natural form is more understandable. Long sentences confuse the reader; shorter ones (not choppy sentences) are usually preferred.

Study the following examples to learn how to overcome three common faults: the clogged sentence, the overburdened sentence, and the too-complex sentence.

The Clogged Sentence

Poor: *Lila Davenport, age 56, of 75 State Street, who told the staff nurses that she had never been hospitalized, and whose husband had died three months ago in the same hospital, was reluctant to sign the consent form that would authorize her pending exploratory surgery.*

Improved: *Lila Davenport was reluctant to sign the consent form for her pending exploratory surgery. The 56-year-old woman told the staff nurses that her husband had died in the same hospital three months earlier.*

The Overburdened Sentence

Similar to the clogged sentence, it is packed with ideas rather than facts.

Poor: *Under the legislature's health plan for the past decade, the proposed new amendment for health professional education now before the Senate Education Committee, and soon to go before the House Education Committee, not only deals with funding for all types of nurse manpower but also for the creation of several new categories of health care technicians.*

Improved: *The health professional amendment being proposed before Congressional committees not only deals with funding for nurses but also for new categories of health care technicians.*

The Too-Complex Sentence

This type of sentence resembles and sometimes combines clogged and overburdened sentences.

Poor: *At the time of the critical nurse shortage during the late 1980's, and because of public concern over the crisis, especially in view of the fact that hospitals were closing units and turning away patients not only in the Northeast but all over the nation, the nursing profession mobilized its leadership to seek long-term solutions and not just immediate answers to this recurring problem in recruitment and retention.*

Improved: *Because of public concern with the nursing shortage of the late 1980's, the profession mobilized its leadership to seek long-term solutions for a recurring problem. As a result of the crisis, hospitals nationwide closed units and turned away patients.*

D. Master Transitional Words and Phrases

Within paragraphs, transitions are words, phrases, or structures that ease an orderly passage from one idea to the next. The term transition simply means "to change." A common way of performing transitions between sentences in a paragraph is to use connectives such as however, therefore, on the other hand, meanwhile, at the same time, then, and afterward.

She accompanied the technician into the patient's room. Afterward, she called the lab to get the blood test results.

Transitional words or phrases at the start of new paragraphs form logical links to the preceding paragraphs. Examples include: on the contrary, as a result, therefore, furthermore, and in addition to. Transitional paragraphs are used to separate, summarize, compare or contrast, and emphasize.

IV

Reduce Redundancy

"Brevity is the soul of wit."

You've heard that one before! The Great Bard knew what he was talking about. One of the first approaches to economical expression is recognizing and eliminating redundant terms. Padding, or the use of unnecessary words or phrases, clutters and obscures meaning. Trim your writing and join the other "word watchers of America." In the following list, the words in *italics* are redundant.

a period of one year
absolutely essential
adequate enough
advanced planning
advanced warning
all-inclusive
attached *hereto*
basic fundamentals
blue *in color*
boxlike *in shape*
complete absence
completely unanimous
connected *together*

consensus *of opinion*
continue *on*
costs *the sum of*
cull *out*
each *and every*
early *on*
eliminate *completely*
enclosed *herewith*
end result
endorse *on the back*
entirely completed
exact same
extremely minimal

few *in number*
final outcome
foreseeable future
full and complete
future plans
future prospects
generally speaking
habitual custom
handsome *looking*
important essential
in my *best* judgment
intradermal skin tests
    (eliminate either
    intradermal or skin)
male prostate gland
many *in number*
modern hospital *of today*

my *own* autobiography
off *of*
past experience
past history
personal opinion
pre planning
reason *why*
recur *again*
research *study*
revert *back*
round *in shape*
serious crisis
small *in size*
spell out *in detail*
temporary reprieve
true facts
unexpected surprise

V

Say What You Mean

A. Steer Clear of Euphemisms

Euphemisms are words or phrases designed to avoid using harsh, blunt, or offensive terms. Substitute the "real thing." Here are some examples:

Euphemism	Substitute
concerned	worried, perplexed
deceased, passed away	died, dead
experience discomfort	hurt
frustrate	annoy, disappoint
inappropriate	wrong, untimely, inept
negative evaluation	disapproval
noncompliant	defiant
nonperformance	failure, neglect
not comfortable with	disagree, dislike
terminate	die, end

B. Substitute Sensitive Language

Accentuate the positive when using language to describe disabled persons; emphasize them rather than their disability. Try to incorporate words and phrases that convey the dignity of the individual.

Some examples of preferred words and phrases follow:

developmentally disabled	persons with AIDS
disabled	persons with cerebral palsy
hearing impaired	persons with disabilities
mentally/emotionally disabled	persons with paraplegia
mentally restored	seizure
mobility impaired	visually impaired
multihandicapped	wheelchair-user
nondisabled	

Poor: *Ms. Davis is a crippled woman confined to a wheelchair.*

Improved: *Ms. Davis is a woman with a disability who uses a wheelchair.*

Poor: *The victims in the rehabilitation program were afflicted with a variety of problems.*

Improved: *Participants in the rehabilitation program included individuals with disabilities due to cerebral palsy, war injuries, and alcohol abuse.*

VI

Eliminate Triteness

Trite expressions or cliches are familiar combinations of words, often used quotations, and worn-out figures of speech. They should be replaced. Here are some examples:

acid test
after all is said and done
age before beauty
all that glitters is not gold
all work and no play
(with) bated breath
better late than never
blue in the face
blushing bride
bolt from the blue
breathe a sigh of relief
bright and shining faces
brown as a berry
budding genius
chip off the old block
clear as a bell
cool as a cucumber
cradle of the deep

dead as a doornail
diamond in the rough
dull thud
fast and furious
few and far between
(the) finer things of life
get off your high horse
green with envy
heart of gold
humble origin
irony of fate
it stands to reason
know-how
leaps and bounds
method in your (his, my)
  madness
ominous silence
path to success

proud possessor
quiet as a mouse
rears its ugly head
road of life
tired but happy
think tank
(the) time of my life

sadder but wiser
sick as a dog
slow as molasses
sly as a fox
smart as a whip
work like a Trojan
wine, women, and song

VII

Know Your Prefixes
and Suffixes

Compound words cause many writing and editing problems.
Are they closed or hyphenated? Two separate words? Are they
treated differently when used as a noun than when used as an
adjective? The list below highlights many of the common prefixes and suffixes.

Here are some principles to follow although exceptions exist:

1. Hyphenate when the compound word is used as an adjective, to avoid confusing the reader, as in *fast-moving train.*

2. Hyphenate if a prefix ends in a vowel and the word that
   follows begins with the same vowel, as in *anti-inflammatory, pre-eminent, pre-exist.*

3. Hyphenate if the word that follows is capitalized, as in
   anti-American, post-Monday, post-March.

4. Hyphenate to join double prefixes, as in *sub-subparagraph.*

5. Hyphenate co- when forming a noun, adjective, or verb
   that refers to an occupation or status, as in *co-chairperson.*

6. Do not hyphenate words formed with the prefix non.

7. Do not hyphenate words formed with the suffix <u>wise</u> when they mean "in the direction of" or "with regard to."
8. Do not hyphenate words formed with the suffix <u>like</u> unless the letters would triple, as in *shell-like.*

Omission of examples indicates that hyphens are generally not used. If in doubt, consult a dictionary.

Prefixes: Affixes before a Word to Produce a Derivative Word

ante
ante-Christianity

antebellum
antedate
antediluvian
anteroom

anti
anti-American
anti-inflammatory
anti-inflation
anti-intellectual

antihypertensive
antisocial
antitoxin
antitrust

bi
biennial
bifocal
bilateral
bilingual
bipartisan
bivalent
biweekly

by
bylaw
byline
bypass
byproduct

co-
co-author
co-chairperson
co-editor
co-host
co-op
co-sponsor
co-worker

coeducation
coexist
cooperate
coordinate

cross
cross-country
cross-examine
cross-purpose
cross-reference
crossbred

crosscut
crosstown

dis
disabled
disaffection
disservice
dissuade

extra
extracranial
extracurricular
extramarital
extraterrestrial

half
half-baked
half-hour
half-life
half-truth
halfhearted
halftime
halfway
half brother
half dollar
half size

hyper
hypercritical
hyperemia
hyperphysical
hyperspace

in
in-group
in-house
in-law
inbound

infield
inpatient

mid
mid-America
mid-Atlantic
mid-1990
mid-80's
midlife
midsemester
midstream
midwest

multi
multidisciplinary
multifaceted
multilateral
multimillionaire

non
non-aligned
non-controversial
nonpartisan
nonviolent
nonworking

over
overachiever
overdue
overeager
overrate
override
oversensitive

post
post-bellum
post-mortem
postbaccalaureate
postdate

postdoctoral
postgraduate
postoperative

pre
pre-exist
pre-election
pre-establish
pre-Hellenic

prearrange
preconference
preheat
premalignant

pro
pro-American
pro-environment

proactive
progovernment
prorated

re
re-emphasize
re-establish
re-use

reconsider
rethink
reunify

self
self-acting
self-address
self-defeating
self-employ
self-evident

semi
semi-independent
semi-invalid

semiannual
semifinal
semiofficial

sub
subaverage
subcommittee
subcontract
subtotal

super
superagency
supercharge
superhighway
superpower
supertanker

trans
trans-Atlantic
trans-configuration
trans-dichloro-ethylene

transcontinental
transcutaneous
transsexual

un
un-American

unarmed
unbelievable
unnecessary
unsolved
unsterile

under
underdog
underestimate
underrepresented
underused

wide	wide-open
wide-angle	widesought
wide-awake	widespread
wide-eyed	

Suffixes: Affixes at the End of a Word to Produce a Derivative Word

in
break-in
cave-in
walk-in
write-in

like
shell-like
bill-like
catlike
lifelike

off
send-off
stop-off
cutoff
playoff
standoff
takeoff

over
carryover
changeover
makeover
rollover
turnover

out
cop-out
fade-out
fallout
pullout
turnout
walkout

up
close-up
follow-up
breakup
buildup
checkup
markup

wise
clockwise
healthwise
taxwise

VIII

Watch Your Spelling

Writers need to be meticulous about their spelling when preparing any written work. Don't be hampered by spelling errors, which can be a source of irritation particularly to editors and teachers. Careless language means a careless person. When in doubt, always use a dictionary.

Here is a listing of words that are commonly misspelled in professional writing:

accommodate
acknowledgment
acute care (noun),
    acute-care (adjective)
aegis
aftercare
afterward (not afterwards)
all right (not alright)
ambiance
amid (not amidst)
among (not amongst)
anonymity
bed linen (two words)
beginning
benefited, benefiting

bona fide
byproduct
canceled
cannot
caregiver
case mix
case mix index
caseload
child rearing (noun)
    child-rearing (adjective)
commitment
committable
committed
computer-assisted instruction
consensus

corollary
corroborate
cost-effective (adj.)
course work
credentialing
criterion, criteria
cross section (noun),
    cross-section (adj.)
data bank
database
day care
decision making (noun),
    decision-making (adj.)
degree-granting
dichotomy
downtime
eighth
embarrassed
enforce
entry level (noun),
    entry-level (adj.)
existence
extended care facility
field work
fieldwork (military usage
    only)
flow chart (preferred)
    (noun)
flow-chart (verb)
foci (plural)
focused
forehead
fulfillment
fundraising (preferred)
grassroots
hands-on
handwashing
holistic

home health aide
home health care
immediately
impatient
in-depth (adj.)
in-house (adj.)
joint faculty
judgment
Kardex (proper noun)
knowledge
leisure
liaison
licensure
lifeless
life-sized
life-style
life-support (adj.)
line-item (adj.)
long-standing
low-key
lower-division
melee
naive
naivete
ninety
nonfat
nonmember
non-nurse
nonprofit
occurred
ongoing
on-line
on-site
outnumber
outpatient
paradigm
parallel
policymaker, policymaking

printout
privilege
programmed
programming (preferred)
prophecy (noun),
   prophecies (plural)
prophesy (verb)
prostate
questioning, questioned
questionnaire
quid-pro-quo
range-of-motion
rank and file (noun)
   rank-and-file (adj.)
recurrence
respondent
rhythm
role playing (noun)
second-guess
seize
self-care
shining
shortfall
short-run (adj.)
side effect

skeptic
spreadsheet
step-down (adj.)
synonymous
tenure-track (adj.)
third party
thus (not thusly)
toward (not towards)
tragedy
time-and-motion
traveling, traveled (preferred)
under way (adv.)
   underway (adj.)
upper-division
well-being
well-baby clinic
word processing (noun),
   word-processing (adj.)
work force
workload
workout
workplace
workup
write-off
write-up

IX

Use Computers to Augment Your Skills

No modern stylebook would be complete without mentioning the capability of computer programs to augment your writing skills. Although new and more sophisticated software is continually in the works, you need to assess what the growing body of editorial programming can and cannot do for you. The most telling observation is that computer software in this area has many positive aspects, but it is *not* a substitute for a good stylebook, dictionary, or English composition text.

Nevertheless, computer users can capitalize on a variety of word processing add-on products with components not found in standard word-processing programs. Although most software has a limited capacity for checking grammar, spelling, and readability, and for containing dictionaries and a thesaurus, the stand-alone programs appear to be more comprehensive than those equipped with a word processor. The majority are available for both IBM (DOS and Windows) and Macintosh users.

Below is a summary of what you can expect.

Grammar Checkers

This software analyzes words within the context of the sentences in which they are used. The computer highlights errors and suggests corrections. Most programs have "pulldown" help menus for rules on grammar and style. In some cases, you can adapt the grammar checker to your particular field of writing, such as business, fiction, legal, scientific, technical, and so on.

Some editorial software programs will create mark-up copy with your changes. Study the document and then revise after the software has completed its analysis. With other programs, you can make changes as you go along. Keep in mind that you have the option of ignoring any of the suggestions since your judgment may dictate otherwise.

Each software program is unique, but almost all that are currently available can identify and correct problems in the following areas:

abbreviations
adverb and adjective usage
archaic usage
colloquial expressions
double negatives
end-of-sentence prepositions
jargon
long sentences

passive voice
pronoun cases
punctuation and spelling
  errors
redundancies
split infinitives
subject-and-verb agreement
wordiness

Many grammar checkers (and some word processors) also analyze a document, giving statistics as to percentage of uses of passive voice, readability and writing level, sentence and paragraph length, and other areas.

Among the editorial software programs are *Correct Grammar* (Word Star International); *Grammatik 5* (Reference Software International); and *Right Writer* (Que Software). Health professionals will be interested in a medical edition of *Correct Grammar*, marketed by Williams & Wilkins. This program combines *Correct Grammar*'s regular grammar checking, style, and spelling features with a comprehensive *Stedman's Medical Dictionary/25 medical word list*. It also will check your style against the *AMA Manual of Style, 8th Edition*, the *Publication Manual of the American Psychological Association*, and *Medical Style and Format* by Dr. Edward J. Huth.

Dictionaries and Spell Checkers

Databases of both medical and general words are now available. Whereas some only highlight and correct spelling or usage, others provide detailed definitions. An electronic thesaurus can respond promptly to synonyms for words. Also on the market are programs on foreign language words and on famous quotations.

Based on the *American Heritage Dictionary* (office edition), *Definitions Plus!* functions as an electronic on-line dictionary. *Stedman's Definitions,* produced by Williams & Wilkins, provides access to 40,000 medical definitions. This software will enable you to check usage and spelling, as well as to locate the exact meaning of a word or phrase. As a spell checker, *Stedman's/25 Plus* contains 20,000 new trade and generic drug names, 15,000 additional medical words, and a capitalization element to check eponyms, trade names, abbreviations, and chemical symbols.

A handy reference for computer users is *The Random House Encyclopedia,* which offers a host of information arranged in a hierarchy of categories from the arts to the sciences. It differs from the book version in that the program includes several ways to use the contents—an outline view showing a vertical format, or a graphic view in a series of scrollable columns.

Outliners

These powerful tools help to organize and reorganize thoughts and information. Although useful in preparing presentations and organizing large word processing documents, this software is highly complex. One such product is *Grandview* (Semantic Corporation).

File Conversion

Converting a document from one file format to another often becomes necessary in light of the many available word processors.

Most programs can perform this skill, but you may encounter a format that cannot be translated. Standard file conversion programs, however, can often preserve most of the formatting of a document that would normally be lost if you converted a file to an ASCII format. Among the programs are *Software Bridge* and *Word for Word Professions* for DOS, Windows, and Macintosh.

Conclusion

From the above review of current editorial software, you will note that many attractive features are available. Supporters revel in the utility of the technology and are delighted with the prospect of the computer's "catching all my writing errors."

At the same time, such remarks may be shortsighted. Although helpful, most programs do have their imperfections. With a grammar checker, for example, a computer often flags errors where none exists. It also fails, in many cases, to find the correct subject and verb of a sentence. Furthermore, there is a tendency to call every complex sentence a "run on."

Spell checkers, too, have their limitations. It is not unusual for a program to highlight a word, indicate that it is not in the dictionary, and suggest alternatives. What this really means is that the word in question does not exist in that particular software's dictionary!

As a health professional eager to write well, you should use wisely the kinds of editorial software described herein. Be mindful that such programs offer no promise of enhancing your creativity or assisting in the development of your own style. View these aids primarily as adjuncts to the writing skills you must acquire through practice and the use of sound print resources on composition and style. These are the best ways to *learn to be your own editor.*

X

References for Further Reading

American heritage dictionary of the English language (3rd ed.). (1992). Boston: Houghton Mifflin.

American Psychological Association. (1984). *Publication manual of the American Psychological Association* (3rd ed.). Washington, DC: Author.

Associated Press. (1987). *Associated Press stylebook and libel manual: The journalist's bible.* Menlo Park, CA: Addison-Wesley.

Chapman, R. L. (1992). *Roget's international thesaurus* (5th ed.). New York: HarperCollins.

Dillard, A. (1990). *The writing life.* New York: HarperCollins.

Duncan, A. (1989). *A dictionary for nurses.* New York: Springer.

Fondiller, S. H. (1992). *The writer's workbook.* New York: National League for Nursing.

Gehle, Q., & Rollo, D. (1987). *Writing essays: A process approach.* New York: St. Martin's.

Gordon, K. E. (1983). *The well-tempered sentence.* New York: Ticknor & Fields.

Gordon, K. E. (1984). *The transitive vampire.* New York: Times Books.

Houghton Mifflin English. (1984). *Grammar and composition.* Boston: Houghton Mifflin.

Lambeth, D. (1976). *The golden book on writing.* New York: Viking Penguin.

Lewis, J. (1982). *The New York Times manual of style and usage.* New York: Random House.

Raimer, A. (1992). *Grammar trouble spots. An editorial guide for students.* New York: St. Martin's.

Strunk, W. J., & White, E. B. (1979). *The elements of style.* (3rd ed.). New York: Macmillan.

The Chicago manual of style (13th ed.) (1982). Chicago: University of Chicago Press.

Warriner, J. E., & Griffiths, F. (1977). *English grammar and composition* (Heritage ed.). New York: Harcourt Brace Jovanovich.

Webster's new world college dictionary (3rd ed.) (1989). Englewood Cliffs, NJ: Prentice-Hall.

XI

Common Proofreader's Marks

Mark	Explanation	Example
‖	Align/No indent	‖ Cleveland is
᷍ᴸⁱ	Boldface	⁍ᵧ <u>Cleveland</u>
x	Broken letter	Clevelᛪnd ⅋
e/	Correction	Clevᛁland e/
⌒	Close up space	Cleve⌒land
⊆	Capital letter	c̲leveland
≡	Capitalize	<u>Cleveland</u>
ᴘ	Delete	Cleveᵍland
▢	Indent 1 em	▢ Cleveland is the
▭	Indent 2 ems	▭ Cleveland is the
▭▭	Indent 3 ems	▭▭ Cleveland is the

Mark	Explanation	Example
⌃2	Inferior (subscript) figures (symbols)	CO_2 CO_2
⧣	Insert space	ClevelandⱯthe ⧣
⌄	Insert apostrophe	Clevelands riverfront
⌃	Insert a comma	ClevelandⱯOhio
£/ɟ/	Insert brackets	ClevelandⱯOhioⱯ £/ɟ/
⟨/⟩/	Insert parentheses	ClevelandⱯOhioⱯ ⟨/⟩/
⊙	Insert a period	Cleveland, Ohio⊙
⌃	Insert information	ClevⱯland e⌃
⌄ ⌄	Insert quotation marks	⌄I like Cleveland⌄ ⌄ ⌄
stet	Let it stand	Cleveland is the (stet)
‿	Less space	Cleve‿land
⌣/	Lower	Cleveland ⌣is/
lc	Lowercase letter	Cleveland /s lc
lc	Lowercase letters	CL/EVELAND lc
⊏	Move left	⊏| Cleveland
⊐	Move right	⊐Cleveland |
¶	New paragraph	the last. ⌃Cleveland is the ¶
no ¶	No new paragraph, run in	the last. ⊐ ⊏Cleveland is the no ¶

Mark	Explanation	Example
⌒	Raise	Cleveland ⌐is⌐
ital	Set in italics	<u>Cleveland</u> ital
rom	Set in roman type	Cleveland rom
＝	Small capitals	<u>Cleveland</u>
4⋁	Superior (superscript) figures (footnotes)	Cleveland is the largest 4⋁
tr	Transpose	Cleveland⌐the⌐is⌐ tr
tr	Transpose in order	Cleveland capital the is not
wf	Wrong font	Cleveland wf

Index

Other Books of Interest from NLN Press

Book Title	Pub. No.	Price	NLN Member Price
☐ The Writer's Workbook By Shirley Fondiller	14-2470	$23.95	$20.95
☐ On Nursing: A Literary Celebration By Margretta Styles & Patricia Moccia	14-2512	29.95	26.95
☐ On Nursing: A Literary Celebration Collector's Leatherette-Bound Edition	14-2513	54.95	49.95
☐ The NLN Guide to Undergraduate RN Education From the NLN Center for Career Advancement	41-2524	19.95	17.95
☐ Scholarships and Loans for Nursing Education 1993-1994	14-1964	14.95	12.95
☐ Computers in Small Bytes: The Computer Workbook By Irene Joos, Nancy Whitman, Marjorie J. Smith, and Ramona Nelson	14-2496	25.95	22.95
☐ Directory of Educational Software for Nursing By Christine Bolwell	41-2405	87.95	79.95